ATI TEAS Practice Tests Version 6:

600 Test Prep Questions
for the TEAS 6 Exam

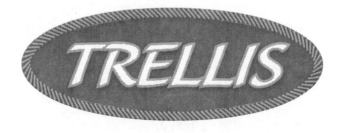

Contents

ATI TEAS 6 Exam Breakdown

Congratulations! You've decided to enter the world of nursing. You're in for a long journey ahead, but you've chosen an excellent profession. We wish you the best of luck in your new career.

The first order of business is to successfully pass the Test of Essential Academic Skills (TEAS). The TEAS is an admissions exam used by many nursing schools to assess potential students and their likely future success. Nursing students who take the TEAS must be prepared to complete reading, math, science and English language sections on the exam. The table below illustrates the question breakdown and time limits for the TEAS test.

Section	Time	Questions Asked	Questions Scored
Reading	58 minutes	48 questions	42 questions
Mathematics	51 minutes	34 questions	30 questions
Science	66 minutes	54 questions	48 questions
English Language	34 minutes	34 questions	30 questions
TOTAL	**209 minutes**	**170 questions**	**150 questions**

Note: While you're required to answer 170 questions, only 150 will be scored. The remaining 20 are used for internal purposes only.

TEAS Reading
The TEAS reading section evaluates your reading comprehension. The questions in this section involve reading passages and answering questions associated with main ideas, details, inferences and question stems.

TEAS Mathematics
The TEAS mathematics section evaluates your mathematical knowledge. The questions in this section involve working with numbers, mathematical operations, measurement and data.

TEAS Science
The TEAS science section evaluates your scientific understanding. This section is by far the most important and extensive section for the TEAS exam...after all, you are working to become a nurse! The questions in this section involve answering questions related to anatomy, biology, physical science and scientific reasoning.

TEAS English Language
The TEAS English language section evaluates your English language skills. The questions in this section involve the correct usage of grammar, context and punctuation.

The TRELLIS TEAS 6 Practice Workbook

This TEAS 6 practice workbook is designed to be used either as a stand-alone or as a supplemental study aid in preparation for the TEAS 6 exam. The practice questions on the following several pages have been fully updated by our team of TEAS experts for the new TEAS version 6 test.

For your convenience, this book consists of three different types of TEAS 6 practice tests:
- Basic practice tests
- Intermediate practice tests
- Advanced practice tests

Because of this arrangement, the practice questions will be increasingly more challenging as you proceed from the basic to intermediate to advanced practice tests. Our advice is to work through the basic practice tests, then intermediate, and finally advanced.

So, you know the overall structure of the TEAS 6 test, and you know how to use this TEAS 6 practice workbook to achieve the greatest benefit. Now, it's time to get some practice in.

Good luck, and let's get started.

BASIC PRACTICE TEST: SCIENCE

1- What causes the motion of the tectonic plates on the Earth's surface?

    A. The rotation of the Earth

    B. The difference in density between the Earth's surface plates and the Earth's mantle layer

    C. Convection currents in the Earth's mantle layer

    D. The force of gravity acting to draw high elevation land masses toward the much lower elevation seafloors

2- What is the explanation for the fact that the same side of the moon always faces the Earth?

    A. The moon does not rotate around a central axis

    B. The moon completes one full central-axis rotation in the same amount of time that it completes one full orbit of the Earth

    C. The moon faces one side to the Earth at night and the other side during the day

    D. The moon completes one rotation in exactly the same amount of time that is required for the Earth to complete one full rotation

3- On the surface of the Earth, an object will experience a force of gravity that does which of the following?

    A. Increases as the velocity of the object increases

    B. Is directly proportional to the object's mass

    C. Is twice as great as the force of gravity that the object would experience if it were exactly one Earth radius in distance above the Earth's surface

    D. Is one half as great as the force of gravity that the object would experience if it were exactly one Earth radius in distance above the Earth's surface

4- What is the difference between alternating current (AC) and direct current (DC) in an electrical circuit?

    A. The direction that electrons flow through a circuit reverses at a fixed rate of electron flow direction per unit time for alternating current. The direction that electrons flow through a circuit remains constant for direct current.

    B. Direct current electrons enter and leave the circuit at a single site. Alternating current electrons enter a circuit at one site but leave the circuit at another site.

    C. Alternating current electrons switch between two voltage values at a fixed rate per unit time while traveling in a circuit. Direct current electrons always have an unchanging voltage value while traveling in a circuit.

    D. There are two opposite simultaneous flow directions for electrons in an alternating current circuit but only one flow direction in a direct current circuit.

5- If two different species are members of the same order, what two items must they then also be members of?

    A. Genus and Class

B. Genus and Phylum
C. Family and Division
D. Class and Division

6- If a sample substance consists entirely of only one element, what must all of the individual atoms of the sample substance have?

A. The same atomic mass
B. The same number of nucleons
C. The same number of neutrons
D. The same atomic number

7- In SI units, what is one joule (J) equivalent to?

A. 1 newton (N) times 1 meter (m)
B. 1 kilogram (kg) times 1 meter squared (m^2) divided by one second squared (s^2)
C. 1 watt (W) divided by 1 meter (m)
D. 1 kilogram (kg) times 1 meter squared (m^2) divided by one second (s)

8- What is the general structure of a typical eukaryotic cell membrane?

A. A single outer lipid molecule layer
B. A bilayer of phospholipid molecules
C. A sugar-phosphate molecule outer layer and collagen fibril inner layer
D. A cellulose molecule outer layer and glycoprotein inner layer

9- What is the pH range that includes the pH of a 5×10^{-3} M aqueous solution of hydrochloric acid (HCl)?

A. 3.5 to 4.0
B. 5.0 to 6.0
C. -3.5 to -4.5
D. 3.0 to 2.0

10- A young boy is swinging a 0.5-kg ball tethered to a 0.5-meter-long rope around himself in a circular path in the horizontal plane (parallel to the ground). At any given instant in time, the ball has a tangential velocity with an unchanging scalar magnitude of 20 meters per second ($m-s^{-1}$). Ignoring any other forces acting on the ball, such as gravity, wind resistance or friction, what is the force acting on the ball through the rope during the time that the ball is undergoing this type of motion?

A. 50 N
B. 20 N
C. 250 N
D. 400 N

$F_c = m \cdot v^2 / r$

$.5 kg \cdot 20 / .5m$

11- What are the two physiological responses that will occur due to activation of the sympathetic nervous system?
    A. Pupil constriction and bronchial dilation
    B. Pupil dilation and bronchial constriction
    C. Pupil dilation and bronchial dilation
    D. Pupil constriction and suppression of digestion

12- What would be the likely long-term effect of a rapid reversal (over approximately 100 to 1000 years) of the Earth's magnetic fields?
    A. A continued normal evolution of the present ecosystem
    B. An abrupt mass extinction followed by a recovery that is typical after previous mass extinctions
    C. No immediate ecological effect but eventual loss of the atmosphere due to the effects of the solar wind
    D. The extinction of all life on Earth permanently

13- What is the energy generated by the sun a result of?
    A. Fission of uranium and plutonium atoms
    B. Fusion of uranium and plutonium atoms
    C. Fission of hydrogen atoms
    D. Fusion of hydrogen atoms

14- An object with a mass m_1 is resting on a flat horizontal frictionless surface. Ignoring the effects of air resistance, what will be the acceleration experienced by the object when a force of 15 N is applied to the object in a horizontal direction?
    A. $15 \text{ N}/m_1$
    B. $m_1/15 \text{ N}$
    C. $(15 \text{ N})(m_1)$
    D. $(15 \text{ n})^2/2m_1$

$F = ma$ $a = F/m_1$

15- A simple circuit consists of a single light bulb that is connected to a single 5-volt (V) battery. If the electrical resistance of the light bulb is 0.25 ohms (Ω), what is the current in amperes (A) in this electric circuit?
    A. 0.05 amperes (0.05 A)
    B. 20 amperes (20 A)
    C. 1.25 amperes (1.25 A)
    D. 1.0 amperes (1.0 A)

16- If a child has a physical trait that is determined by a single gene and that physical trait is not present is the child's biological mother or biological father, then which of the following is true?

A. There is only one allele for that trait's gene.

B. The trait's gene is not a sex-linked gene.

C. The trait's gene likely has two alleles, one that is recessive and one that is dominant.

D. The trait's gene likely has at least three alleles, and all of the alleles are recessive.

17- How many cubic centimeters are equivalent to the volume of a cubic meter?

A. 1000

B. 10,000

C. 100,000

D. 1,000,000

18- At the end of its stellar lifecycle, which of the following will the sun be?

A. White dwarf

B. Neutron star

C. Black hole

D. Red giant

19- What is a way that a light wave differs from a sound wave?

A. A light wave cannot travel through a vacuum

B. A light wave increases velocity when, on Earth, it passes from air into water

C. A sound wave's maximum velocity is less than a light wave's maximum velocity

D. A sound wave cannot change its wavelength

20- An optical instrument that causes incident light rays traveling parallel to its focal axis to converge at a focal point in front of the optical surface could be which of the following?

A. A simple concave mirror

B. A simple convex mirror

C. A simple biconcave lens

D. A simple biconvex lens

21- A ray of light is traveling through a substance that has an index of refraction of 2. The ray then passes through a horizontal interface between the substance with a refractive index of 2 and into a substance that has a refractive index of 3. The light ray enters the substance at an angle less than 90 degrees with respect to the interface. Imagine a perpendicular line is drawn through the horizontal interface at the point that the ray crosses into the substance with a refractive index 3. As the light ray continues on its path, what will it do?

A. Slow down and bend toward the perpendicular line

B. Slow down and bend away from the perpendicular line

C. Speed up and bend toward the perpendicular line

D. Speed up and bend away from the perpendicular line

22- Which of the selections includes the list of three planets that is ranked in increasing size from left to right?

  A. Saturn, Uranus, Jupiter

  B. Mercury, Mars, Venus

  C. Earth, Saturn, Neptune

  D. Mars, Mercury, Saturn

23- What two events each represent physical changes to molecular compounds?

  A. Reduction reactions and oxidation reactions

  B. Evaporation and deprotonation

  C. Reduction reactions and sublimation

  D. Filtration and dilution

24- What would be the atomic mass of the element Helium if it consisted of equal percentages of exactly two isotopes, one with the same number of protons and neutrons and the other with one more neutron than protons?

  A. 2

  B. 3.5

  C. 4.5

  D. 5

25- A chloroplast requires energy in what form to carry out its most important function inside a cell?

  A. Chemical energy derived from the hydrolysis of ATP

  B. Electromagnetic energy derived from the absorption of photons

  C. Chemical energy derived from anaerobic cellular respiration resulting in the conversion of glucose to lactic acid and other chemical products

  D. Energy derived from the concentration gradient of protons across the inner membrane of the chloroplast

26- According to Newton's 3rd law of motion, which of the following is true?

  A. A force is required to change the velocity of an object

  B. A gun will experience a force of magnitude 5 N at the same instant that it fires a 5-g bullet that experiences an initial acceleration of 1000 m/s

  C. No force is required to maintain an object in a circular orbit

  D. The final potential energy of any ideal one body system is always equal to zero

27- Consider a circuit that consists of a power source and three resistors, R_1, R_2 and R_3. The resistance values are R_1 = 10 Ω, R_2 =4 Ω and R_3 =2 Ω. Which of the following connection patterns for some or all of these resistors could result in a total resistance for the circuit of 11 ⅓ Ω?

A. R_2 and R_3 are connected in parallel

B. R_1, R_2 and R_3 are connected in series

C. R_1, R_2 and R_3 are connected in parallel

D. R_1 and R_3 are connected in parallel

28- Atoms in their lowest electron energy state will begin to add electrons to their 3d electron orbitals immediately after they have filled which of the following?

A. 2s orbital

B. 2p orbitals

C. 3s orbital

D. 3p orbitals

29- Three separate objects with three different individual masses and velocities undergo a simultaneous, perfectly elastic collision. The objects' motions are confined to a horizontal frictionless surface. No other forces with the exception of gravity are acting on the objects and there is no air resistance. Which of the following statements is true regarding the objects before and after this collision?

A. The total momentum of the objects has changed after the collision but the total kinetic energy of the objects has remained constant

B. The total momentum and kinetic energy of the objects before and after the collision has not changed

C. The total momentum of the objects remains the same before and after the collision but the total kinetic energy of the objects has changed

D. Both the total momentum and kinetic energy of the objects before and after the collision have changed

30- A weightlifter is holding a 100-kg barbell motionless 2 meters above the ground for 5 seconds. During this 5-second timespan, the weightlifter has done which of the following?

A. Increased his momentum

B. Expended no energy

C. Performed no work on the barbell

D. Converted kinetic energy to potential energy

31- A car is traveling north on a perfectly straight highway. The car's current velocity is 60 miles/hour. The car begins to accelerate at a constant rate of 10 miles/hour². How far north will the car travel over the next 2 hours?

A. 140 miles

B. 150 miles

C. 180 miles

D. 220 miles

32- If the mass of the Earth increased by a factor of 4 and the radius of the Earth increased by a factor of 2, what would happen to the weight of an object on the surface of the Earth?

    A. Increase by a factor of 2

    B. Decrease by a factor of 2

    C. Increase by a factor of 8

    D. Remain unchanged

33- An object has a mass of 1400 kg and a velocity of 1 m/s. Which changes in the mass and/or velocity of the object in the answer options below would result in the largest increase in the object's kinetic energy?

    A. Increase the object's mass by 1000 g

    B. Increase the object's velocity by 1 m/s and decrease its mass by 600 g

    C. Increase the object's velocity by 2 m/s and decrease its mass by 950 g

    D. Decrease the object's velocity by 0,5 m/s and increase its mass by 1050 g

34- What is the angular acceleration, "A_c", of an object in uniform circular motion, where the radius "R" of the circular motion is 2 m and the magnitude of the tangential velocity 'V" is 40 m/s?

    A. $10 \ m/s^2$

    B. $80 \ m/s^2$

    C. $800 \ m/s^2$

    D. $1600 \ m/s^2$

35- The Earth orbits the Sun in a nearly circular path. If M_e = the mass of the Earth, M_s = the mass of the Sun, R_{es} = the radius of the distance between the center of the Earth and the center of the Sun, G = the gravitational constant, and F_g = the force of gravity between the Earth and the Sun, what is an equation that gives the mass of the Earth based on Newton's law of universal gravitation?

    A. $M_e = (F_g)(R_{es})^2/(G)(M_s)$

    B. $M_e = (R_{es})(G)(M_s)/ F_g$

    C. $M_e = (R_{es})^2(M_s)/(F_g)(G)$

    D. $M_e = (F_g)(G)/(R_{es})(M_s)$

36- Two objects, A and B, are traveling at constant velocities directly toward each other on a frictionless horizontal surface. Other than gravity, there are no other forces and no air resistance acting on the two objects. The mass and velocity of object A is: M_A = 1 kg and V_A = 20 m/s. The mass and velocity of object B is: M_B = 2 kg and VB = -30 m/s. When the two objects collide, they stick together and continue to move as a single combined object, "AB". What is the resulting velocity," V_r", of the object AB?

    A. 1 2/3 m/s

    B. 4.5 m/s

C. -10 m/s

D. -13 1/3 m/s

37- What will individual atoms of an element that is a good electrical conductor most likely have?

    A. An atomic number that is less than 10

    B. Valence electron shells that are more the one-half filled

    C. One or more mobile valence electrons per atom

    D. No valence shell electrons

38- A 10-kg object is at rest on a horizontal surface. The surface has a coefficient of static friction of 0.75 with respect to the object. No other forces except for gravity are acting on the object. What is the initial force acting in a horizontal direction required to accelerate the mass at 5 m/s (use 10 m/s^2 for "g" the acceleration of the object due to gravity)?

    A. 50 N

    B. 150 N

    C. 200 N

    D. .500 N

39- In the U.S., standard wall outlet alternating current (AC) is 60 Hz. If this AC begins to flow past a point in a wire beginning at time zero with amplitude of zero amps and increasing to its peak positive amplitude of 1 amp, what will be the current value at this point in the wire at a time 1/120th of a second after time zero?

    A. Zero

    B. 1 A

    C. -1 A (one ampere of current traveling in the opposite direction)

    D. 0.5 A

40- An electric current of 10 A is flowing through a circuit connected to a 20-V battery. What is the total power that is dissipated by all of the resistors this circuit?

    A. 2 coulombs

    B. 200 coulombs

    C. 2 watts

    D. 200 watts

41- In the chemical reaction $CH_4 + 2O_2 \rightarrow 2H_2O + CO_2$, the chemicals H_2O and CO_2 are both what two things?

    A. Reactants and ionic compounds

    B. Reactants and covalent compounds

    C. Products and ionic compounds

    D. Products and covalent compounds

42- Among the choices below, which method would most likely be able to separate a mixture of two isotopes of hydrogen, H^1 consisting of one proton and H^2 consisting of one proton and one neutron?

    A. A chemical reaction with fluorine

    B. A chemical reaction with lithium

    C. A physical separation based on freezing points

    D. A physical separation based on mass

43- A 1-molar aqueous solution of the weak acid HA has a pH of 3.7. What percentage of hydrogen ions in this solution is contributed by the dissociation of water molecules?

    A. greater than 50% but less than 75%

    B. Greater than 75%

    C. Greater than 1% but less than 10%

    D. Less than 1%

44- When a virus infects a eukaryotic cell, which cell organelles are directly required to assemble the copies of the viral proteins?

    A. The Golgi apparatus

    B. Ribosomes

    C. Chloroplasts

    D. Lysosomes

45- If the moon was twice as close to the Earth and completed one orbit of the Earth in exactly the same amount of time that the Earth requires to complete one full rotation on its axis, then which of the following would be true?

    A. High tide height would increase and high tides would occur once per day

    B. High tide height would increase and high tides would occur four times per day

    C. High tide height would decrease and low tides height would increase

    D. There would be no tides on Earth that occur due to the effects of the moon

46- At a movable skeletal joint, what are the ends of the adjoining bones covered by?

    A. Ligaments

    B. Cartilage

    C. Tendons

    D. Muscle fibers

47- What is the most important function of the epiglottis?

    A. Prevention of gastric acid reflux into the lower esophagus

    B. Generation of sound required for speech

    C. Protection of the airway

D. Production of salivary amylase

48- During inhalation, air first passes from the nasal cavity directly to which of the following?
A. Esophagus
B. Pharynx
C. Larynx
D. Primary bronchi

49- What do the pulmonary veins transport?
A. Deoxygenated blood to the right atrium
B. Deoxygenated blood to the left atrium
C. Oxygenated blood to the right atrium
D. Oxygenated blood to the left atrium

50- Which of the following may a person whose blood type is A positive do?
A. Donate blood to a person whose blood type is A negative
B. Donate blood to a person whose blood type is O negative
C. Receive blood from a person whose blood type is AB negative
D. Receive blood from a person whose blood type is O positive

51- What is the primary function of bile during the digestion of food?
A. Break down starch
B. Emulsify fat
C. Acidify the contents of the stomach
D. Break down proteins

52- In the human female reproductive system, where is the endometrial lining located?
A. Ovaries
B. Fallopian tubes
C. Uterus
D. Vagina

53- The cerebellum plays a central role in which of the following?
A. Coordination of movements
B. Processing of visual information
C. Controlling simple reflexes such as the patellar tendon knee jerk reflex
D. Controlling breathing and heartrate

54- What is a difference between the infectious agent that causes strep throat and the infectious agent that causes influenza?

A. The strep throat agent is a virus

B. The influenza agent is susceptible to antibiotics

C. The strep throat agent possesses a nucleus

D. The influenza agent is much less biologically complex than the strep throat agent

55- Which of the following is a heritable disease that is caused by a recessive allele of a single gene?

A. Cystic fibrosis

B. Huntington's disease

C. Mesothelioma

D. Tuberculosis

56- The packaging of substances that are synthesized inside a cell for transport outside of the cell is the primary function of which part of the cell?

A. Lysozymes

B. Centromeres

C. Golgi apparatus

D. Mitochondria

57- For eukaryotic cells, which of the following is true of the separation of sister chromatids?

A. Occurs during mitosis but not during meiosis

B. Occurs during meiosis but not during mitosis

C. Occurs during both mitosis and meiosis

D. Does not occur during normal cell cycles

58- What does a self-sustaining food web require?

A. Autotrophs

B. Omnivores

C. Herbivores

D. Carnivores

59- Which direct rock type transformation is currently occurring at the Earth's surface or within one to two miles beneath the surface of the Earth?

A. Sedimentary to igneous

B. Metamorphic to igneous

C. Sedimentary to metamorphic

D. There are no longer any rock type transformations occurring within the upper two miles of the Earth's crust.

60- What is the gas that comprises approximately 20% of the Earth's atmosphere?

A. Nitrogen

B. Oxygen
C. Carbon dioxide
D. Argon

61- Assuming g = 10 m/s, what is – as close as possible - the minimum amount of power required to raise a 10,000-kg mass 1 kilometer in 100 seconds above the surface of the Earth?

    A. 1000 watts

    B. 100,000 watt

    C. One million watts

    D. Ten billion watts

62- In humans, two alleles for the same gene that are present in the somatic cells of a male parent that follow the law of independent assortment are most likely which of the following?

    A. Dominant alleles

    B. Located on different chromosome pairs

    C. Located on the Y chromosome

    D. Located on separate chromosomes of a chromosome pair

63- What is the sum of all the forces acting on a 50-kg object that has a constant velocity of magnitude 40 m/s?

    A. Zero

    B. 200 N

    C. 2000 N

    D. 40,000 N

64- The amount of energy that the human body can extract from 1 gram of glycogen is closest to the amount of energy the human body can extract from which of the following?

    A. 1 gram of fat

    B. 1 gram of glucose

    C. 2 grams of protein

    D. 3 grams of lactic acid

65- As the distance of a light source from an observer increases, what happens to the apparent light intensity?

    A. Decreases in direct proportion to the square root of the distance

    B. Decreases in direct proportion to the distance

    C. Decreases in direct proportion to the distance squared

    D. Decreases in direct proportion to the distance cubed

66- In the periodic table of the elements, what are the group VIII elements known as?

A. Halides
B. Alkali metals
C. Transition metals
D. Noble gases

67- As the kinetic energy of an object increases, which of the following happens?
   A. Acceleration always decreases
   B. Velocity always increases
   C. Mass always decreases
   D. Density always increases

68- Which of the answer choices describes the effect that hydrogen bonding would have on compounds with low molecular weights?
   A. Increased freezing point
   B. Increased boiling point
   C. Increased acidity
   D. Decreased density in the liquid phase

69- Among the meteorological conditions described below, where are large complexes of cumulous clouds most likely to form?
   A. At the border region of colliding warm and cold fronts
   B. After several days over a stationary front
   C. After several days over a strong high pressure region
   D. After several weeks of very high temperatures in a flat terrain bordered by high mountains on the side of the terrain that first encounters prevailing winds

70- Since the moon orbits the Earth once per lunar month, why do total eclipses of the sun not occur at least once per lunar month?
   A. Because the moon is tidally locked to the Earth
   B. Because the Earth is in orbit around the sun
   C. Because the Earth rotates an average of approximately 28 days for each orbit of the moon around the Earth
   D. Because the Earth's orbit around the sun is not perfectly circular

71- The ovaries in human females, in addition to their reproductive role, are also which of the following?
   A. Participants in the urinary excretory system
   B. Innervated by the sympathetic nervous system
   C. Endocrine glands
   D. Thermoregulatory organs

72- Which of the following statements is true as it relates to all organisms in the plant and animal kingdoms?

A. There are no omnivores that are also autotrophs
B. There are no carnivores that are also scavengers
C. There are no carnivores that are also omnivores
D. There are no detritivores that are also scavengers.

73- How does a metallic vacuum thermos bottle slow the loss of heat from hot liquids to the cooler outside environment?

A. By decreasing radiative heat loss only
B. By decreasing convective heat loss only
C. By decreasing convective and conductive heat loss only
D. By decreasing conductive, convective and radiative heat loss heat.

74- A 60-kg woman is standing in a basket. A frame connected to the basket forms an apex above the woman's head. Attached to the apex is a rope that passes over a frictionless horizontal bar just beneath a supporting 20-meter horizontal structural support. The rope loops over the bar and down to the woman's hands. Assume the woman's strength and endurance are not limiting factors. By simply pulling down on the rope, what is the woman capable of?

A. She cannot pull both herself and the basket upward toward the horizontal bar
B. She can pull both herself and the basket upward toward the horizontal bar if the rope has no coefficient of friction
C. She can pull both herself and the basket upward toward the horizontal bar if the basket weighs more than 60 kg
D. She can pull both herself and the basket upward toward the horizontal bar if the basket weighs less than 60 kg

75- Carbon that is derived from carbon dioxide that did not exist in the Earth's atmosphere at an earlier time is currently being released into the atmosphere by what process or event?

A. Volcanic eruptions
B. Hydroelectric power generation
C. Fossil fuel usage
D. Radioactive decay of boron (B)

76- What is the primary role of dietary fiber in the human digestive process?

A. Absorption of bile acids
B. Mechanical removal of dental plaque
C. Facilitation of bowel movements
D. Detoxification of the small intestine

77- What is the Earth's magnetic field generated by?

    A. The Earth's inner core

    B. The Earth's outer core

    C. Solar radiation

    D. Movement of the Earth's tectonic plates

78- The first appearance of large numbers of macroscopic fossils in the geological record of the Earth marks the end of which geological period?

    A. The Precambrian eon

    B. The Permian era

    C. The Ordovician era

    D. The Silurian era

79- What type of electron orbital is used by atoms to form pi bonds?

    A. S orbitals

    B. P orbitals

    C. SP orbitals

    D. SP_2 orbitals

80- Which of the following is a constant throughout the universe?

    A. The gravitational constant g

    B. The speed of light

    C. The weight of the proton

    D. The matter density of the universe

81- What are the most powerful storm systems on Earth the result of?

    A. Stationary fronts

    B. Low-pressure systems

    C. Warm fronts

    D. High-pressure systems

82- Which are the three major regions of the solar system that contain the highest total mass of asteroids and/or comets?

    A. Asteroid belt, Van Allen belt and Kuiper belt

    B. Oort cloud, asteroid belt and Kuiper belt

    C. Magellanic cloud, Oort cloud, and Van Allen belt

    D. Asteroid belt, Magellanic cloud and Proxima Centauri

83- Which of the following does a normal human gamete always have?

    A. 16 pairs of chromosomes

B. One X and one Y chromosome

C. A total number of 23 unpaired chromosomes

D. 22 pairs of chromosomes

84- In ecology, what is a community defined as?

    A. All of the animals in a geographical isolated region

    B. A species that consists of a single or a few fertile "queen" females and a large number of infertile females living together as a cooperative group

    C. A collection of all interdependent species in a geographical region

    D. A group of human individuals that live and work together for the benefit of all members of the group

85- In humans, what are essential amino acids?

    A. All of the amino acids required to build all of the proteins found in the body

    B. The amino acids required to synthesize neurotransmitters

    C. The amino acids that are only available through dietary intake

    D. The fundamental building blocks for the synthesis of all other amino acids in the body

86- Which of the following does the Earth have, compared to Saturn?

    A. A larger orbital radius of the sun

    B. A slower axial rotation

    C. A lower overall density

    D. A stronger magnetic field

87- Which of the following does the pancreas NOT secrete?

    A. Pepsin

    B. Insulin

    C. Glucagon

    D. Lipase

88- What are persons with a long-standing dietary deficiency of vitamin D most directly at increased risk of?

    A. Scurvy

    B. Atherosclerosis

    C. Osteoporosis (bone demineralization)

    D. Malignant melanoma

89- A man with a mass of 100 kg is standing on a scale in an elevator 100 meters above the surface of the Earth. As the elevator begins to descend, the man observes that, for a brief period of time, his weight decreases by 50% according to the scale upon which he is standing. What could explain this apparent decrease in the man's weight?

    A. The elevator is accelerating downward at 4.9 m/s^2

    B. The elevator is accelerating upward at 9.8 m/s^2

    C. The elevator is moving at exactly half of its terminal velocity through air with a pressure of exactly 1 atmosphere

    D. The elevator has a coefficient of static friction of 0.5

90- If the protons of an atom's nucleus reversed their electric charge but remained exactly the same in every other respect, the atom could exist as a neutrally charged atom if the nucleus was orbited by which electrically bound item?

    A. Neutrons

    B. Neutrinos

    C. Positrons

    D. Quarks

91- Visible light that is emitted from a galaxy that is receding from our galaxy at very high velocity may be detected as what type of electromagnetic energy by observers on the Earth?

    A. Radio waves

    B. Ultraviolet light

    C. X-rays

    D. Gamma rays

92- If a bar magnet consisting of naturally magnetic iron is bisected into two separate pieces at a point perpendicular to its magnetic polar axis, then which of the following is true?

    A. The two pieces will each have a positive and negative magnetic pole

    B. The two pieces will each have neither a positive nor a negative pole

    C. One piece will have two negative magnetic poles and the other will have two positive magnetic poles

    D. One piece will have a positive and a negative magnetic pole and the other will have neither a positive nor a negative magnetic pole

93- What is not a sub classification of the kingdom "Plantae" ?

    A. Bryophyta

    B. Coelenterata

    C. Gymnospermia

    D. Tracheophyta

94- If an atom of an unknown element "X" were to lose 3 protons from its nucleus, what could it represent a conversion of?

A. Oxygen (O) atom to a boron (B) atom

B. Argon (A) atom to an aluminum (Al) atom

C. Potassium (K) atom to a sulfur (S) atom

D. Lithium (Li) atom to a hydrogen (H) atom

95- Among the choices below, in a sample of a crystal consisting of a single pure ionic salt compound, which of the following two elements are most likely to occur in a two-to-one ratio?

A. Magnesium and chlorine

B. Lithium and fluorine

C. Sodium and bromine

D. Calcium and oxygen

96- Where is the ozone layer located In the Earth's atmosphere?

A. Adjacent to and above the thermosphere

B. Adjacent to and above the mesosphere

C. Adjacent to and above the stratosphere

D. Adjacent to and above the troposphere

97- In humans, among the choices below, which is considered the most desirable blood cholesterol profile for a normal young adult?

A. Low HDL and LDL levels

B. High HDL and LDL levels

C. A Low HDL level and a high LDL level

D. A high HDL level and low LDL level

98- Which of the following is true regarding the Fahrenheit temperature scale compared to the Celsius temperature scale?

A. A one-degree increase on the Fahrenheit scale is a larger temperature increase than a one-degree increase on the Celsius scale

B. A one-degree increase on the Fahrenheit scale is a smaller temperature increase than a one-degree increase on the Celsius scale

C. Absolute zero is a larger absolute number on the Celsius scale

D. The boiling point of water is a smaller number on the Fahrenheit scale

99- In the water cycle, "infiltration" is the term used to define which movement of water?

A. As a gas, from the atmosphere, into plants

B. As a gas, from plants, into the atmosphere

C. As a liquid, from the Earth's surface, to underground reservoirs

D. As a liquid, from underground reservoirs, into open bodies of water

100- One of the characteristics that ecologists include in their definition of a biome is that it is a geographical region that does what?

    A. Contains only one apex predator

    B. Shares the same climate

    C. Provides all animal life access to a common water source

    D. Encompasses the entire range of life-sustaining habitats on Earth

INTERMEDIATE PRACTICE TEST: MATHEMATICS

1 – The number of students enrolled at Two Rivers Community College increased from 3,450 in 2010 to 3,864 in 2015. What was the percent increase?

    A. 9%

    B. 17%

    C. 12%

    D. 6%

2 – Find the median in this series of numbers: 80, 78, 73, 69, 100.

    A. 69

    B. 73

    C. 78

    D. 80

3 – Solve this equation: $\sqrt{11 * 44} =$

    A. 36

    B. 24

    C. 18

    D. 22

4 – Amy drives her car until the gas gauge is down to 1/8 full, then she fills the tank to capacity by adding 14 gallons. What is the capacity of the gas tank?

    A. 16 gallons

    B. 18 gallons

    C. 20 gallons

    D. 22 gallons

5 – Which of these numbers is largest?

    A. −345

    B. 42

    C. −17

    D. 3^4

6 – Which of the following is a prime number?

A. 81
B. 49
C. 59
D. 77

7 – The area of a triangle equals one-half the base times the height. Which of the following is the correct way to calculate the area of a triangle that has a base of 6 and a height of 9?

    A. $(6 + 9)/2$
    B. $\frac{1}{2}(6 + 9)$
    C. $2(6 * 9)$
    D. $\dfrac{(6)(9)}{2}$

8 – Calculate the value of this expression: $2 + 6 * 3 * (3 * 4)^2 + 1$

    A. 2,595
    B. 5,185
    C. 3,456
    D. 6,464

9 – If $x \geq 9$, which of the following is a possible value of x?

    A. 2^3
    B. 9
    C. –34
    D. 8.5

10 – Solve this equation: $-9 * -9 =$

    A. 18
    B. 0
    C. 81
    D. –81

11 – Solve this equation: $x = a^2 * a^3$

    A. $x = a$
    B. $x = a^5$
    C. $x = 1$
    D. $x = 0$

12 – Jean buys a textbook, a flash drive, a printer cartridge, and a ream of paper. The flash drive costs three times as much as the ream of paper. The textbook costs three times as much as the flash drive. The printer cartridge costs twice as much as the textbook. The ream of paper costs $10. How much does Jean spend altogether?

A. $250
B. $480
C. $310
D. $180

13 – Which of the following is the smallest possible integer value of x in this equation: $x > 3^2 - 4$

A. 3
B. 5
C. 6
D. 7

14 – In the graduating class at Emerson High School, 52% of the students are girls and 48% are boys. There are 350 students in the class. Among the girls, 98 plan to go to college. How many girls do not plan to go to college?

A. 84
B. 48
C. 66
D. 72

15 – A cell phone on sale at 30% off costs $210. What was the original price of the phone?

A. $240
B. $273
C. $300
D. $320

16 – Seven added to four-fifths of a number equals fifteen. What is the number?

A. 10
B. 15
C. 20
D. 25

17 – If the sum of two numbers is 360, and their ratio is 7:3, what is the smaller number?

A. 72
B. 105
C. 98
D. 108

18 – Alicia must have a score of 75% to pass a test of 80 questions. What is the greatest number of questions she can miss and still pass the test?

A. 20
B. 25

C. 60

D. 15

19 – Carmen has a box that is 18 inches long, 12 inches wide, and 14 inches high. What is the volume of the box?

A. 44 cubic inches

B. 3,024 cubic inches

C. 216 cubic inches

D. 168 cubic inches

20 – The lines in the diagram below are

A. Parallel

B. Perpendicular

C. Acute

D. Obtuse

21 – Find the area.

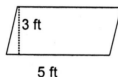

3 ft

5 ft

A. 16 square feet

B. 7.5 square feet

C. 15 square feet

D. 30 square feet

22 – Which of these numbers is largest?

A. 5/8

B. 3/5

C. 2/3

D. 0.72

23 – It took Charles four days to write a history paper. He wrote 5 pages on the first day, 4 pages on the second day, and 8 pages on the third day. If Charles ended up writing an average of 7 pages per day, how many pages did he write on the fourth day?

A. 11

B. 8

C. 12
D. 9

24 – What is the approximate area of the portion of the square that is not covered by the circle?

4 ft

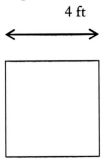

A. 4.14 square feet
B. 3.44 square feet
C. 6.25 square feet
D. 5.12 square feet

25 – Which of the following is equivalent to the equation: $\dfrac{5}{mp} \div \dfrac{p}{4}$

A. $\dfrac{5p}{4mp}$

B. $\dfrac{20}{mp^2}$

C. $\dfrac{20mp}{4p}$

D. $\dfrac{4mp}{5p}$

26 – Danvers is 8 miles due south of Carson and 6 miles due west of Baines. If a driver could drive in a straight line from Carson to Baines, how long would the trip be?
A. 8 miles
B. 10 miles
C. 12 miles
D. 14 miles

27 – Lourdes rolls a pair of 6-sided dice. What is the probability that the result will equal 10?
A. 1/36
B. 2/36

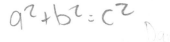

C. 3/36

D. 4/36

28 – Four friends plan to share equally the cost of a retirement gift. If one person drops out of the arrangement, the cost per person for the remaining three would increase by $12. What is the cost of the gift?

A. $144

B. $136

C. $180

D. $152

29 – What is the factorial of 5?

A. 25

B. 5 and 1

C. 120

D. 125

30 – Which digit is in the thousandths place in this number: 1,234.567

A. 1

B. 2

C. 6

D. 7

31 – What is the mode in this set of numbers: 4, 5, 4, 8, 10, 4, 6, 7

A. 6

B. 4

C. 8

D. 7

32 – Which of the following numbers is a perfect square?

A. 5

B. 15

C. 49

D. 50

33 – Amanda makes $14 an hour as a bank teller, and Oscar makes $24 an hour as an auto mechanic. Both work eight hours a day, five days a week. Which of these equations can be used to calculate how much they make together in a five-day week?

A. (14 + 24) * 8 * 5

B. $\dfrac{14 + 24}{(8)(5)}$

C. (14 + 24) (8 + 5)

D. 14 + 24 * 8 * 5

34 – The population of Mariposa County in 2015 was 90% of its population in 2010. The population in 2010 was 145,000. What was the population in 2010?

    A. 160,000

    B. 142,000

    C. 120,500

    D. 130,500

35 – What is the sum of 1/3 and 3/8?

    A. 3/24

    B. 4/11

    C. 17/24

    D. 15/16

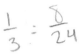 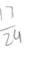

36 – In four years, Tom will be twice as old as Serena was three years ago. Tom is three years younger than Serena. How old are Tom and Serena now?

    A. Serena is 28, Tom is 25

    B. Serena is 7, Tom is 4

    C. Serena is 18, Tom is 15

    D. Serena is 21, Tom is 18

37 – A rectangle's length is three times its width. The area of the rectangle is 48 square feet. How long are the sides?

    A. Length = 12, width = 4

    B. Length = 15, width = 5

    C. Length = 18, width = 6

    D. Length = 24, width = 8

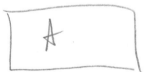

38 – Which of the following is the prime factorization of 24?

    A. 24 = 8 * 3

    B. 24 = 2 * 2 * 2 * 3

    C. 24 = 6 * 4

    D. 24 = 12 * 2

39 – x is a positive integer. Dividing x by a positive number less than 1 will yield:

    A. A number greater than x

    B. A number less than x

    C. A negative number

    D. An irrational number

40 – Solve this equation: $x = 8 - (-3)$
   A. $x = 5$
   B. $x = -5$
   C. $x = 11$
   D. $x = -11$

41 – Which of the following statements is true?
   A. The square of a number is always less than the number.
   B. The square of a number may be either positive or negative.
   C. The square of a number is always a positive number.
   D. The square of a number is always greater than the number.

42 – Marisol's score on a standardized test was ranked in the 78th percentile. If 660 students took the test, approximately how many students scored lower than Marisol?
   A. 582
   B. 515
   C. 612
   D. 486

43 – Sam worked 40 hours at d dollars per hour and received a bonus of $50. His total earnings were $530. What was his hourly wage?
   A. $18
   B. $16
   C. $14
   D. $12

$$530$$
$$-50$$
$$\overline{480} = 12$$
$$40$$

44 – Solve for r in this equation: $p = 2r + 3$
   A. $r = 2p - 3$
   B. $r = p + 6$
   C. $r = \dfrac{p+3}{2}$
   D. $r = \dfrac{p-3}{2}$

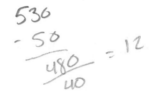

45 – What is the least common multiple of 8 and 10?
   A. 80
   B. 40
   C. 18
   D. 72

46 – Solve this equation: $x = -12 \div -3$

A. $x = -4$
B. $x = -15$
C. $x = 9$
D. $x = 4$

47 – Convert the improper fraction 17/6 to a mixed number.

A. $2\frac{5}{6}$

B. $3\frac{1}{6}$

C. 6/17

D. $3\frac{5}{6}$

48 – What value of q is a solution to this equation: $130 = q(-13)$

A. 10
B. –10
C. 1
D. 10^2

49 – Find the value of $a^2 + 6b$ when $a = 3$ and $b = 0.5$.

A. 12
B. 6
C. 9
D. 15

50 – If the radius of the circle in this diagram is 4 inches, what is the perimeter of the square?

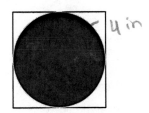

A. 24 inches
B. 32 inches
C. 64 inches
D. 96 inches

51 – Solve for x in the following equation: $x = \frac{3}{4} * \frac{7}{8}$

A. 7/8
B. 9/8

C. 10/12

D. 21/32

52 – Which of the following is equal to half a billion?

    A. 50,000,000

    B. 500,000,000

    C. 500,000

    D. 50,000,000,000

53 – Which of the following represents the relationship between x and y in this table?

x	y
0	7
3	13
5	17
7	21
8	23

    A. $y = x + 7$

    B. $y = 4x + 1$

    C. $y = 2x + 10$

    D. $y = 2x + 7$

54 – When you add two numbers, the sum is 480. If the ratio of the two numbers is 5:1, what is the smaller number?

    A. 60

    B. 70

    C. 72

    D. 80

$$x + 5x = \frac{480}{5}$$
$$\frac{}{5}$$

$$x + 5x = 480$$

55 – In a high school French class, 45% of the students are sophomores, and there are 9 sophomores in the class. How many students are there in the class?

    A. 16

    B. 18

    C. 20

    D. 22

56 – What is the perimeter of this figure?

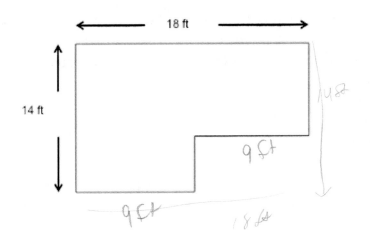

A. 64 ft
B. 72 ft
C. 84 ft
D. 96 ft

57 – What exponent should replace the question mark: $15{,}200 = 1.52 * 10^{?}$
  A. 2
  B. 3
  C. 4
  D. 5

58 – Which of the following is equal to 0.0065?
  A. $6.5 * 10^{-2}$
  B. $6.5 * 10^{-3}$
  C. $6.5 * 10^{-4}$
  D. $6.5 * 10^{-5}$

59 – At a lunch cart, there are 2 orders of diet soda for every 5 orders of regular soda. If the owner of the lunch cart sells 112 sodas a day, how many are diet and how many are regular?
  A. 28 diet, 84 regular
  B. 32 diet, 80 regular
  C. 34 diet, 82 regular
  D. 36 diet, 84 regular

60 – What is the greatest common factor of 48 and 64?
  A. 4
  B. 8
  C. 16
  D. 32

61 – Two rectangles are proportional; that is, the ratio of length to width is the same for both rectangles. The smaller rectangle has a length of 8 inches and a width of 3 inches. The larger rectangle has a length of 12 inches. What is the width of the larger rectangle?
   A. 4 inches
   B. 4.5 inches
   C. 6 inches
   D. 8.5 inches

62 – The average weight of five friends (Al, Bob, Carl, Dave, and Ed) is 180 pounds. Al weighs 202 pounds, Bob weighs 166 pounds, Carl weighs 190 pounds, and Dave weighs 192 pounds. How much does Ed weigh?
   A. 180 pounds
   B. 172 pounds
   C. 186 pounds
   D. 150 pounds

63 – Find the value of the expression $x^2 + y^3$ when $x = -3$ and $y = -5$
   A. –116
   B. 134
   C. –134
   D. 116

64 – Alan commutes 18 miles to work. Bob's commute is 4 miles shorter. Ted's commute is 6 miles shorter than Bob's. Rebecca's commute is shorter than Alan's but longer than Bob's. Which of the following could be the length of Rebecca's commute?
   A. 12 miles
   B. 14 miles
   C. 15 miles
   D. 18 miles

65 – Of the patients admitted to an ER over a one-week period, 14 had heart attacks, 15 had workplace injuries, 24 were injured in auto accidents, 12 had respiratory problems, 21 were injured in their homes, and 34 had other medical problems. What percent of these patients had respiratory problems?
   A. 10%
   B. 12%
   C. 15%
   D. 18%

66 – The ratio of female to male nurses in a hospital is 9:1. If there are 144 female nurses, how many male nurses are there?

A. 12
B. 14
C. 16
D. 18

67 – A square 8 inches on a side is cut into smaller squares 1 inch on a side. How many of the smaller squares can be made?

A. 8
B. 16
C. 24
D. 64

68 – Which of the following statements is true?

A. 2 is the only even prime number.
B. The largest prime number less than 100 is 89.
C. The greatest common factor of 24 and 42 is 4.
D. The least common multiple of 8 and 6 is 48.

69 – Which of the following falls between 2/3 and 3/4?

A. 3/5
B. 4/5
C. 7/10
D. 5/8

70 – What is the value of this expression if $a = 10$ and $b = -4$:

$$\sqrt{2a + b^2}$$

A. 6
B. 7
C. 8
D. 9

$2(10) + (-4)^2$

$20 + 16$

$\sqrt{36}$

71 – What is the slope of the line in this graph?

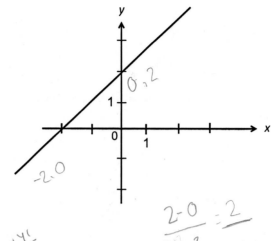

A. 1
B. –1
C. 2
D. –2

72 – Kevin has his glucose levels checked monthly. These are the results:

January	February	March	April	May	June	July
98	102	88	86	110	92	90

In which month was his glucose level equal to the median level for these seven months?

    A. January
    B. March
    C. April
    D. June

73 – A committee studying an economic issue includes 3 state legislators, 6 state employees, and several members of the public. If one person is selected at random from the committee, the probability that the person will be a state legislator is 1/5. How many of the members of the committee are members of the public?

    A. 5
    B. 6
    C. 8
    D. 9

74 – Mark will randomly choose 2 different letters from the word MINUTE. If the first letter he chooses is an M or an N, what is the probability that the next letter he chooses will be an M or an N?

    A. 1/4
    B. 1/5

C. 1/6

D. 1/3

75 – At Pleasantville College, the ratio of female to male students is exactly 5 to 4. Which of the following could be the number of students at the college?

    A. 8,200

    B. 2,955

    C. 3,500

    D. 3,105

76 – Which of the following is equivalent to 60% of 90?

    A. 0.6 * 90

    B. 90 ÷ 0.6

    C. 3/5

    D. 2/3

77 – The perimeter of a rectangle is 24 inches, and the ratio of the length to the width is 2:1. What is the area of the rectangle?

    A. 60 square inches

    B. 18 square inches

    C. 32 square inches

    D. 48 square inches

78 – The three teams with the best records in the division are the Bulldogs, the Rangers, and the Statesmen. The Bulldogs have won nine games and lost three. The Rangers have won ten games and lost two. The Statesmen have also won ten games and lost two. Each team has one game left before the playoffs. The Bulldogs will be playing the Black Sox, and the Rangers will be playing the Statesmen. The team with the best record will win a spot in the playoffs. Which of the following statements is true?

    A. The Statesmen will definitely be in the playoffs.

    B. The Bulldogs will definitely not be in the playoffs.

    C. The Rangers will definitely not be in the playoffs.

    D. The Statesmen will definitely not be in the playoffs.

79 – Which of the following is equivalent to $1.34 * 10^5$?

    A. 134,000

    B. 13,400

    C. 1,340,000

    D. 13,400,000

80 – If $a = -4$, what is the value of $a^3 - a - 2$?

A. 66
B. −62
C. 68
D. −66

81 – Brian pays 15% of his gross salary in taxes. If he pays $7,800 in taxes, what is his gross salary?
    A. $52,000
    B. $48,000
    C. $49,000
    D. $56,000

82 – Which of the following expressions is not equivalent to the others?
    A. $4^2 * 5 * 3$
    B. $2^3 * 15 * 2$
    C. $3^3 * 5 * 2$
    D. $2^3 * 10 * 3$

83 – On a roulette wheel, there are 37 pockets numbered 0 through 36. On any given spin, what is the probability that the ball will land on an odd number?
    A. 1/2
    B. 1/37
    C. 18/37
    D. 17/37

84 – Solve the following equation: $y^5 \div y^3$
    A. y
    B. y^2
    C. y^3
    D. y^4

85 – What is the smallest positive integer that is evenly divisible by 5 and 7 and leaves a remainder of 4 when divided by 6?
    A. 35
    B. 70
    C. 105
    D. 140

86 – Which of the following can be the lengths of the sides of a triangle?
    A. 1,2,4
    B. 2,4,8
    C. 2,3,4

D. 4,5,9

87 – In her retirement accounts, Janet has invested $40,000 in stocks and $65,000 in bonds. If she wants to rebalance her accounts so that 70% of her investments are in stocks, how much will she have to move?
    A. $33,500
    B. $35,000
    C. $37,500
    D. $40,000

88 – Eight identical machines can produce 96 parts per minute. How many parts could 12 of these machines produce in 3 minutes?
    A. 144
    B. 288
    C. 256
    D. 432

89 – The average of 25, 35, and 120 is 10 more than the average of 40, 45, and what number?
    A. 60
    B. 65
    C. 70
    D. 76

90 – There are 3 more men than women on the board of directors of the Big Box Retail Company. There are 13 members on the board. How many are women?
    A. 3
    B. 4
    C. 5
    D. 6

91 – Which linear equation is depicted by this graph?

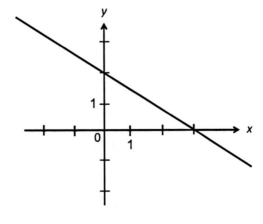

A. y = 2x + 1
B. y = –2/3x + 2
C. y = –3x + 1
D. y = 3x + 2

92 – What is the value of x in the following equation:

$$\frac{4}{9}x - 3 = 1$$

A. 9
B. 8
C. 7
D. –4½

93 – Solve this system of equations:

$$x - 3y = 15$$
$$x + 2y = 25$$

A. $x = 24, y = 6$
B. $x = 21, y = 2$
C. $x = 28, y = 8$
D. $x = 25, y = 4$

94 – If the y-intercept of the depicted line is reduced by 1, what would be the slope of the resulting line?

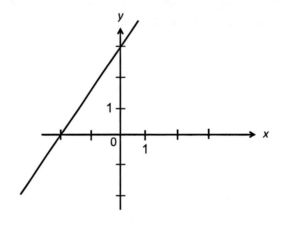

A. –1
B. –2
C. 2
D. 1

95 – Solve this system of equations:

$$x - 2y = 8$$

$$2x + 6y = 36$$

    A. $x = 16, y = 2$

    B. $x = 18, y = 4$

    C. $x = 12, y = 2$

    D. $x = 26, y = 1$

96 – Solve this equation: $2x^2 + 9x + 4 = 0$

    A. $x = 2$ or 6

    B. $x = -1/2$ or -4

    C. $x = -2$ or -4

    D. $x = -1/2$ or 2

97 – Solve this equation: $4x^2 + 12x + 5 = 0$

    A. $x = 4$ or -4

    B. $x = -2$ or 4

    C. $x = -\dfrac{1}{4}$ or $-\dfrac{1}{2}$

    D. $x = -\dfrac{1}{2}$ or $-2\dfrac{1}{2}$

98 – What is the sum of all prime numbers less than 25?

    A. 100

    B. 89

    C. 77

    D. 101

99 – Convert $2\dfrac{1}{3}$ to an improper fraction.

    A. 5/3

    B. 3/7

    C. 7/3

    D. 8/3

100 – The product of two numbers is 6 more than their sum. Which of these equations describes this relationship?

    A. $xy + 6 = x + y$

    B. $xy = x + y + 6$

    C. $xy = 6x + 6y$

    D. $xy = x + y - 6$

101 – Consider a rectangle with a length of 8 and a width of 6. What must be the length of each side of a square that has the same perimeter as the rectangle?

    A. 5
    B. 6
    C. 7
    D. 8

INTERMEDIATE PRACTICE TEST: SCIENCE

1- Bronchial epithelial cell membranes possess which of the following?

    A. microvilli
    B. cillia
    C. flagella
    D. dendrites

2- Emulsification of fats requires _____ and occurs in the _____.
Which of the following correctly completes the statement above?

    A. amylase; stomach;
    B. bile; stomach
    C. amylase; small intestine
    D. bile; small intestine

3- In immune functions involving T-helper cells, the T-helper cell most likely engages in which of the following?

    A. phagocytosis
    B. cell lysis
    C. circulating antibody production
    D. intercellular membrane binding

4- In a normal human, once blood is pumped out of the heart , which of the following statements is always true?

    A. It passes through capillaries before returning to the internal chambers of the heart
    B. It has been fully oxygenated.
    C. It immediately enters the aorta
    D. It travels to the lungs before returning to the heart

5- Oxygen enters the circulatory system during

    A. inspiration only
    B. inspiration and the interval between inspiration and expiration only
    C. the interval between inspiration and expiration and during expiration only
    D. continuously throughout the entire respiratory cycle

6- The integrative functions of the nervous system requires which of the following?

    A. Sensory input

    B.   hormonal regulation

    C. spinal cord reflexes

    D. effector cells

7- The duodenum releases which of the following biologically active proteins?

    A. pepsinogen and CCK

    B. CCK and secretin

    C. secretin and trypsinogen

    D. trypsinogen and pepsinogen

8- Which of the following is NOT a capacity of the human innate immune system?

    A. phagocytosis of foreign cells

    B. stimulation of fever

    C. production of antibodies

    D. the release of and response to cytokines

9- Which of the following correctly describes the relative anatomical positional relationship between two anatomical structures in a normal human adult?

    A. The heart is ventral to the esophagus.

    B. The scapula is proximal to the vertebral column.

    C. The kidneys are medial to the abdominal aorta.

    D. The urinary bladder is rostral to the pancreas.

10- In humans, urea is produced in which of the following locations?

    A. the liver

    B. the kidney

    C. the pancreas

    D. red blood cells

11- In humans, which of the organs listed below does NOT receive supplies of both oxygenated and deoxygenated blood?

    A. the lungs

    B. the heart

    C. the liver

    D. the large intestine

12- In humans, which of the skeletal muscles listed below are more often than not under involuntary rather than voluntary control?

    A. the masseters

B. the diaphragm
C. the biceps
D. the tongue

13- In humans, the majority (>50%) of water obtained through oral intake is absorbed into the body through which of the following?
    A. the oral mucosa and the esophagus
    B. the esophagus and the stomach
    C. the small intestines
    D. the large intestines

14- Which of the following cell types secrete perforins?
    A. liver parenchymal cells
    B. natural killer (NK) cells
    C. T-helper cells
    D. vascular endothelial cells

15- In humans, which of the following is true regarding dietary intake of proteins?
    A. It does not occur in individuals who are strict vegetarians
    B. It must include a variety of proteins that consist of all 20 amino acids required for for protein synthesis in the body
    C. inadequate intake during childhood development can lead to the disease kwashiorkor.
    D. breakdown begins when protein reaches the ileum of the small intestine.

Kwashiorkor - inadiquete amant of protein in diet.

16- Among the choices below, which pair of taxonomic categories of organisms are in separate domains?
    A. Eubacteria and Archaebacteria
    B. Fungi and Plantae
    C. Animalia and Protista
    D. Fungi and Protista

17- An absolute requirement for continual adaptation of a species to occur through natural selection is described in which of the following statements?
    A. Mutations in the somatic cells of the fertile members of the species must be able to occur.
    B. Mutations in the germ line cells of the fertile members of the species must be able to occur.
    C. Sister chromatids must be capable of exchanging DNA segments before the completion of meiosis I
    D. Sister chromatids must be capable of exchanging DNA segments before the completion of meiosis II

18- For all biological nucleic acids, a nucleotide is composed of which of the following three components?

    A. a carboxylic acid, a nitrogenous base and a pentose sugar

    B. an amino acid , a hexose sugar and a nitrogenous base

    C. a phosphate group, a pentose sugar and a nitrogenous base

    D. a phosphate group, a hexose sugar and an amino acid

19- Which of the following is a true statement regarding fundamental differences between eukaryotic and prokaryotic cells?

    A. Some, but not all, prokaryotic cells have cell walls, but no eukaryotic cells have cell walls.

    B. Some, but not all, prokaryotic cells have ribosomes, but all eukaryotic cells have ribosomes.

    C. Some, but not all, eukaryotic cells have nucleoids, but all prokaryotic cells have nucleoids

    D. Some, but not all, eukaryotic cells have chloroplasts, but no prokaryotic cells have chloroplasts.

Eukaryotic: Plants, Fungi Single Celled, Animals
Prokaryotic: Without Nucleus - bacteria

20- Which of the following cellular organelles do not possess an outer encapsulating organellar membrane?

encapsulating: enclosed

    A. mitochondria

    B. ribosomes

    C. chloroplasts

    D. nuclei

21- which of the following is true regarding the relationship between a complete segment of mRNA and the gene from which the mRNA segment was transcribed?

    A. The mRNA segment base sequence is identical to the DNA gene base sequence

    B. The mRNA segment base sequence is identical to the complementary DNA strand segment of the gene base sequence

    C. The mRNA segment base sequence is identical to the complementary DNA strand segment of the gene base sequence except that adenine is substituted for thymine in the mRNA base sequence

    D. The mRNA segment base sequence is identical to the complementary DNA strand segment of the gene base sequence except that uracil is substituted for thymine in the mRNA base sequence

22- The gastrulation stage of human fetal development is characterized by which of the following?

    A. Individual tissue layers begin to form

    B. The four fundamental cell types begin to differentiate

    C. The first multipotent stem cells begin to appear

    D. The first individual organs begin to function.

23- The interphase stage of a normal somatic cell cycle consists of which three sub-phases?

    A. prophase, G1 and G2

B. G1, G2, and cytokinesis

C. G1, S and G2

D. G1, S and prophase

24- During the metaphase I stage of meiosis, which of the following events occurs at the metaphase plate?

A. Homologous tetrad pairs align

B. individual tetrads align

C. individual chromatids align

D. homologous chromatid pairs align

25- During photosynthesis, what is the total number of oxygen molecules produced for each molecule of glucose (C6H12O6) that is synthesized?

A. 2

B. 6

C. 12

D. 24

$$6CO_2 + 6H_2O \longrightarrow C_6H_12O_6 + 6O_2$$

26- In human cells, which of the following statements correctly states a true principle of the processing of genetic information?

A. A single, unique sequence of genes codes for a single unique protein

B. A single, unique three-base codon will code for only one single, unique type of amino acid.

C. A single unique protein can only be coded for by a single, unique sequence of codons

D. A single unique protein can only be coded for by a single, unique sequence of of DNA bases.

27- By a strict genetic definition, perfectly identical twins must have _____ .
Select the answer choice that completes the statement above.

A. identical phenotypes only

B. identical genotypes only

C. both identical genotypes and phenotypes

D. either identical genotypes or identical phenotypes

phenotype: characteristics from interaction with environment.

28- In the reaction $H_2CO_3 \longrightarrow HCO_3^- + H^+$, if H_2CO_3 if HCO_3^- is a strong base which of the following is true?

A. H_2CO_3 is a strong acid

B. H_2CO_3 is a weak acid

C. H_2CO_3 is a weak base

D. H_2CO_3 is a strong base

29- The largest fraction of energy that the earth receives from the sun is in the form of which of the following?

    A. kinetic energy of electrons
    B. kinetic energy of neutrons
    C. electromagnetic energy
    D. chemical energy

30- Which of the following has the greatest gravitational potential energy?

    A. a 5 kg mass, at rest, 10 m above the surface of the earth
    B. a 5 kg mass, free-falling, with a current velocity of 10 m/s, 5 m above the surface of the Earth
    C. a 2 kg mass, at rest on the floor of an open vertical shaft, 30 m below the surface of the earth
    D. a 50 kg mass at the instant that it is propelled directly upward with a velocity of 10 m/s

31- An organized functional collection of adipose cells is considered to be which of the following

    A. epithelial tissue   Fat
    B. connective tissue
    C. a syncytium
    D. a gland

32- In chemical reactions where a catalyst participates, the catalyst-------of the reaction by ------of the reaction

    A. increases the efficiency of the reaction; increasing the activation energy
    B. increases the efficiency of the reaction; decreasing the activation energy
    C. increases the rate of the reaction; increasing the activation energy
    D. increases the rate of the reaction; decreasing the activation energy

33- Which of the following is the correct electron configuration for a neutral neon atom in its lowest electron energy state?

    A. 1s2 2s2 2p6
    B. 1s2 2s2 3s2 3p4   1s2
    C. 2s2 2p2 3s2 3p2 3d2
    D. 6s2 2p2

34- In biological chemical systems, an increase in the activity of an enzyme indicates that which of the following has occurred?

    A. The enzyme has increased its optimum functional pH range
    B. The enzyme has increased its optimum functional temperature range
    C. The enzyme has increased its effect on the rate of a chemical reaction
    D. The enzyme has increased the total number of reactions that it is capable of catalyzing.

35- Which of the following lists three substances in DECREASING order of pH value, beginning with the substance with the highest pH on the left?
- A. sulphuric acid, vinegar, water
- B. ammonia, blood, orange juice
- C. water, ammonia, sulphuric acid
- D. vinegar, water, orange juice

36- If an alkane with 6 carbon atoms is converted to an alkyne with 6 carbon atoms, what is the change in the number of hydrogen atoms contained in the alkane compared to the alkyne?
- A. The alkane contains 4 less hydrogen atoms than does the alkyne.
- B. The alkane contains 2 less hydrogen atoms than does the alkyne.
- C. The alkane contains 2 more hydrogen atoms than does the alkyne.
- D. The alkane contains 4 more hydrogen atoms than does the alkyne.

37- which of the following is the site a site of steroid hormone production?
- A. the pancreas *Peptide hormone*
- B. the adrenal gland
- C. the thyroid *Peptide hormones*
- D. the thymus *T cell maturation*

38- In the unbalanced oxidation-reduction reaction $CH4 + O2 ---> CO2 + H2O$, which answer choice below shows the correct, balanced half-reaction for oxygen?
- A. $O2 ---> 2O- + 2e-$
- B. $2O2 + 8e- ---> 4O-2$
- C. $4H+ + 2O ----> 2H2O+$
- D. $CH4 + O2 ---> 1/2CO2 + 1/2H2O$

$CH4 + O2 \rightarrow CO2 + 2H2O$

$C=1$
$H=4/4$
$O=2/4$

$C=1$
$O=2\times4$
$H=2\times4$

39- A sample of liquid bromine ($Br2$) is in an open contained at a pressure of 1 atm and temperature of 20C. As heat is applied to the sample at a constant rate, which of the following will occur beginning at the moment when the bromine sample reaches its boiling point?
- A. The liquid bromine density will increase at a constant rate.
- B. The temperature of the liquid bromine will remain constant.
- C. The volume of liquid bromine that is converted to bromine gas will increase at a constantly increasing rate.
- D. The liquid bromine density will decrease at a constant rate.

40- Water molecules in the liquid state will have____ intermolecular bonding compared to the intermolecular bonding of water molecules in the solid state.
Which of the following correctly completes the statement above?
- A. the same type of
- B. stronger

C. a different type of

D. no

41- Which of the taxonomic classification category pairs listed below begin with the broader category followed by the more specific category?

    A. order; phylum

    B. family; class

    C. class; order

    D. genus; family

42- In a single chromosome___

    Which of the answer choices correctly completes the statement above?

    A. every DNA strand contains genes

    B. there are always two copies of every gene

    C. every functional gene can be transcribed into a mRNA molecule

    D. there are at least 2 alleles for every gene

43- Which of the sequences listed in the answer choices show the correct RNA transcript of the DNA sequence listed below?

    DNA: AGC TAC CCG

    RNA: ___ ___ ___

Uracil Replaces Thymine

    A. TCG ATG GGC

    B. UCG AUG GGC

    C. TCG UTG GGC

    D. CTA GCA AAT

44- Ribosome construction occurs in which of the following locations inside of a cell?

    A. rough endoplasmic reticulum

    B. peroxisomes

    C. lysosomes

    D. nucleoli

45- In terms of processing of genetic information, ribosomes are to proteins as _____ is/are to DNA

    Which of the following completes the analogy shown above?

    A. amino acids

    B. codons

    C. RNA polymerase

    D. DNA polymerase

46- In double-stranded DNA, one strand is called the "sense" strand and the other is called the "anti-sense" strand. Which of the following occurs during replication of double-stranded DNA?

A. The sense strand is completely replicated before replication of the antisense strand begins.

B. The antisense strand is completely replicated before replication of the sense strand begins.

C. Either the sense or the antisense is replicated before replication of the complementary strand begins.

D. Replication of both strands occurs simultaneously.

47- During mitosis, spindle fibers connect which of the following structures?
   A. centromeres and chromosomes
   B. centrosomes and chromosomes
   C. sister chromatids
   D. homologous chromosomes

48- Which of the following correctly describes a role of chlorophyll in living organisms?
   A. transport of oxygen molecules
   B. absorption of sunlight
   C. oxidation of carbon dioxide
   D. production of ATP

49- What are the two general structural categories of nitrogenous bases in nucleic acids?
   A. purines and pyrimidines
   B. thymines and uracils
   C. nucleotides and nucleosides
   D. pyrimidines and hydroxy-ureas

50- Among the choices below, which is the most accurate approximation of the error rate during the replication of DNA that occurs BEFORE any corrective error activities occur.
   A. 1 base error per 1000 genes
   B. 1 base error per 1x10 to the 6 genes
   C. 1 base error per 1x10 to the 6 bases
   D. 1 base error per 1x10 to the 12 bases

51- In some genetic diseases, the disease allele "D" and the normal gene "d" can produce three possible phenotypes. the DD genotype results in severe disease, the Dd genotype results in mild-to-moderate disease, and the dd genotype results in no disease. What is the term for this type of phenotypic pattern of expression?
   A. copenetrance
   B. incomplete penetrance
   C. codominance
   D. incomplete dominance

52- Which of the following is the velocity of an object with a mass of 10 kg mass with a kinetic energy

of 125 joules?
- A. 0.5 m/s
- B. 1.25 m/s
- C. 2.5 m/s
- D. 5.0 m/s

53- Which of the following ratios is closest to 1.0?
- A. the electron charge magnitude to the proton charge magnitude
- B. the proton mass to the neutron mass
- C. the proton charge to the neutron charge
- D. the electron mass to the neutron mass

54- Which of the following statements is true regarding the measurable properties of atoms?
- A. An element's atomic number may be a fractional, rather than a whole number value.
- B. No element's atomic number is larger than the element's atomic mass.
- C. Every individual atom of an element always has the same number of neutrons.
- D. Atoms containing the same number of neutrons but different numbers of protons are isotopes of the same element.

55- In human adults, compared to the other most general types of tissue, which tissue type usually has the highest regenerative capacity?
- A. connective
- B. epithelial
- C. muscle
- D. nervous

56- Among the choices below, during a complete cardiac cycle, which anatomical region experiences the lowest peak blood pressure?
- A. the left atrium
- B. the right ventricle
- C. the pulmonary artery
- D. the left ventricle

Left & Right - thick wall High blood pressure
Ventricle
Pulmonary artery Connected to
left & Right = thin wall low Right ventricle
Atrium B.P.

57- The region(s) of the respiratory airway system that experiences the highest concentration of carbon dioxide is/are the _____.
Select the answer choice that correctly completes the statement above.
- A. left and right main bronchi airspaces
- B. bronchiolar airspaces
- C. alveolar airspaces
- D. tracheal airspace

alveoli - CO_2 diffusing out of Blood Stream

58- Stimulation of the _____ nervous system will most likely result in _____ .

    Select the answer choice that correctly completes the statement above.

      A. sympathetic; decreased bloodflow to the skeletal muscles

      B. central; increase blood flow to digestive tract

      C. parasympathetic; increased peristalsis

      D. central; decreased release of norepinephrine

59- A sudden inability of a human body to produce which of the following will result in chemical injury to the duodenal epithelium of that body?

      A. CCK

      B. Trypsin

      C. Pepsin

      D. Secretin

60- Which of the following is the term for the process where white blood cells move out of a blood vessel and then into the surrounding tissue?

      A. diaphoresis

      B. diapedesis

      C. chemotaxis

      D. facilitated diffusion

61- Which of the following are contents of the dorsal body cavity?

      A. the pharynx and the larynx

      B. the kidneys and the urinary bladder

      C. the brain and the spinal cord

      D. the heart and the lungs

62- The circulatory system participates in thermoregulation by which of the following mechanisms?

      A. vasoconstriction and vasodilation

      B. transport of triglycerides from the liver to adipose tissue

      C. alterations in the permeability of vascular walls to water

      D. alterations in the blood flow rate to the kidneys

63- Which of the following events occurs during contraction of the diaphragm?

      A. Carbon dioxide is expelled from the lower airways.

      B. The thoracic cavity increases its volume.

      C. The lumen of the esophagus is closed at the junction of the entrance to the stomach.

      D. The pupils of the eyes dilate

64- A dense collection of neuron cell bodies located outside of the central nervous system is referred to as which of the following?

A. a synapse

Neurons outside of Nervous System

B. a nucleus

C. a nerve tract

D. a ganglion

65- The absorption of vitamin B12 from the intestines into the body requires which of the following substances secreted by cells located in the stomach?

A. intrinsic factor

B. factor V

C. acetyl coenzyme- A

D. cyclic adenosine monophosphate (cAMP)

66- Passive immunity can be aquired through which of the following processes?

A. vaccination with a killed virus

B. vaccination with a live but weakened form of a virus

C. transfusion of a series of small amounts of Rh positive blood to an Rh negative recipient over a several week period

D. consumption of breast milk

67- Atoms of which element will have a total of 15 electrons in their electron shells when they have a net charge of -3?

A. phosphorous (P)

B. magnesium (Mg)

C. argon (Ag)

D. lithium (Li)

68- In all catalyzed reactions, the catalyst ('s) ____ .

Select the answer choice that correctly completes the statement above.

A. is always an enzyme

B. does not form intermolecular bonds with the participants of the reaction

C. is present in an equal number of catalytic units before the beginning of and after the completion of the catalytic reaction

D. activity is unaffected by the pH of the chemical environment in which the catalyzed reaction occurs

69- Assume a fluoride ion has a complete n=1 electron shell and a completely empty n=2 electron shell. Assume also that all electrons are added to the lowest available electron subshell. Based on this information only, which of the following statements MUST be true?

A. After the first electron is added, the effective nuclear charge that each additional added electron experiences is progressively less than that experienced by the previously added electrons.

B. Only after the 2s orbital is filled, the effective nuclear charge that each additional added electron experiences is progressively less than that experienced by the previously added electrons.

C. Only after the 2s orbital is filled and after one electron is added to each of the 2p orbitals, is the effective nuclear charge that each additional added electron experiences progressively less than that experienced by the previously added electrons.

D. Every electron added to the n=2 level electron shell experiences exactly the same effective nuclear charge.

70- Which of the following atoms, in its lowest electron energy state, has a higher second ionization energy compared to the second ionization energy of a potassium (K) atom in its lowest electron energy state?

A. sodium (Na)

B. calcium (Ca)

C. rubidium (Rb)

D. magnesium (Mg)

71- In bacterial cells, the function of pili is which of the following?

A. cell motility

B. Intercellular transfer of DNA

C. structural support at the cell membrane/cell wall interface

D. intracellular transport of vesicle-packaged substances

72- Among the choices below, at a pressure of 1 atm, which is the temperature where a sample of pure water will have the highest density?

A. -10.0 C

B. -1.0 C

C. 4.0 C

D. 101.0 C

73- if an enzyme can catalyze both the forward reaction: A + B ---> C + D and the reverse reaction as well, which of the following is most likely true?

A. The enzyme has a substrate binding site at at least two physically separated locations.

B. the enzyme's net activity will be zero

C. the enzyme's activity for the reverse reaction will progressively increase to a maximum level as the concentrations of C and D increase

D. The three dimensional structure of the enzyme is bilaterally symmetrical

74- In a comparison between magnesium (Mg) and sulfur (S) atoms, which of the following is true with regard to atomic radius and electronegativity?

A. A neutral magnesium atom's atomic diameter is greater than and electronegativity is less than the atomic diameter and electronegativity of a neutral sulfur atom

B. A neutral magnesium atom's atomic diameter and electronegativity are greater than the atomic diameter and electronegativity of a neutral sulfur atom

C. A neutral magnesium atom's atomic diameter is less than and electronegativity is greater than the atomic diameter and electronegativity of a neutral sulfur atom

D. A neutral magnesium atom's atomic diameter and electronegativity are less than the atomic diameter and electronegativity of a neutral sulfur atom

75- The phosphorus reserves of the body are predominantly stored in which of the following?
   A. mitochondria
   B. liver
   C. bone
   D. the thyroid gland

76- which of the following pairs of different organs are responsible for maintaining blood pH within a very narrow optimum range?
   A. the pancreas and the liver
   B. the liver and the lungs
   C. the lungs and the kidneys
   D. the kidneys and the pancreas

77- Which answer choice identifies the types of DNA error repair mechanisms that correct mutations in germline cells during meiosis?
   A. proofreading and mismatch repair only
   B. proofreading and excision repair only repair only
   C. excision repair and mismatch repair only
   D. proofreading, mismatch repair and excision repair

78- The log of the concentration of H+ ions in a solution is equal to which of the following?
   A. the pH of the solution
   B. the negative log of the pH of the solution
   C. the pH of the solution multiplied by negative 1
   D. The solution pH divided by the H+ ion concentration of the solution

79- What is the general chemical formula for an alkene?
   A. C_nH_{2n+2}
   B. C_nH_{2n}
   C. C_nH_n
   D. C_nH_{n-2}

80- Among the following molecules, which one contains covalent bonds with the LOWEST polarity?

A. CH_4
B. NH_3
C. H_2O
D. HCl

81- Which of the following is not included as a possible modern taxonomic classification of an organism?
    A. Prokaryote
    B. Aves
    C. Canis
    D. Ursidae

82- The latent heat of a substance is related to which of the following?
    A. phase transitions
    B. reaction rates
    C. acidity
    D. combustion

83- In a solid sample of a transition metal element, the elemental atoms will _____ .
Which of the following correctly completes the statement above?
    A. form a rigid crystalline structure
    B. be either oxidized or reduced in equal numbers
    C. be either positively charged or negatively charged in equal numbers
    D. donate valence electrons to a collective valence electron level

84- $HCl_{(aq)} + KOH_{(aq)} \rightarrow$ _____ + _____
which of the following completes the reaction shown above?
    A. $ClOH$; KH
    B. ClH^{2+}; KO^{2-}
    C. KCl; H_2O
    D. KOH^{3+}; $Cl-$

85- Among the choices below, which has the lowest electrical conductivity?
    A. boron
    B. silicon
    C. aluminum
    D. selenium

86- Which of the following is most likely a PRODUCT of a biological fermentation reaction?
    A. O2
    B. glucose

C. CO2

D. HCl

87- Which of the following are the least likely to be directly involved in a cell-mediated immune response?

    A. T-Helper cells

    B. B-cells

    C. natural killer cells

    D. cytotoxic T-cells

88- Which of the following is the Punnett square derived ration for the frequency of heterozygous genotype offspring "Tt" resulting from two heterozygous parents compared to heterozygous offspring resulting from one homozygous parent and one heterozygous parent?

    A. 1 to 1

    B. 1 to 2

    C. 2 to 3

    D. zero

89- Which of the following identifies the units of heat of vaporization?

    A. degrees Celsius and mass

    B. energy and degrees Celsius

    C. energy and mass

    D. volume and degrees Celsius

90- In immune system activities requiring a T-helper cell function the, T-helper cell is most likely directly engaged in which of the following?

    A. phagocytosis

    B. cell lysis

    C. circulating antibody production

    D. intercellular membrane receptor binding

91- By definition two different species cannot _____ .

Which of the following correctly completes the statement above?

    A. share the same ecological niche

    B. belong to the same genus

    C. interbreed

    D. produce fertile offspring

92- If an object with mass "m" is at rest at a height "h" above the surface of the earth, what would be the velocity of the object if all of the object's gravitational potential energy were completely converted to kinetic energy?

A. mgh

B. $h/4g^2$

C. $(2gh)^{1/2}$

D. $(mgh)^2/4$

93- The element _____ serves a direct critical function in the human _____ system.
Which of the following correctly completes the statement above?

A. Iodine; endocrine

B. Iron; nervous

C. Copper; digestive

D. Selenium; nervous

94- Which of the following is the scientific definition of a "light-year"?

A. The amount of sunlight that fall upon the earth in 1 year

B. the distance that light travels in a vacuum in 1 year

C. the subjective time that would elapse for a person who is traveling at the speed of light for one year relative to a stationary observer

D. the total daylight hours experienced by a region of the earth at the equator over a 1 year period.

95- Which of the following describes the anatomical site where the majority of lymphatic fluid is returned to the cardiovascular circulation?

A. at the junction of the thoracic duct and the superior vena cava

B. at the junction of the spleen and the splenic veins

C. at capillaries surrounding lymph nodes

D. at the capillaries of intestinal epithelial villi and intestinal villi lacteals.

96- In ecological terminology, a tropical rainforest is most precisely defined as being which of the following?

A. a zone

B. a biome

C. a terrarium

D. a habitation

97- The smallest unit of matter that consists of different atomic elements that are chemically bonded is

A. a substance

B. a crystal

C. a molecule

D. an ion

98- The majority of atmospheric oxygen is produced by which of the following?

    A. burning of fossil fuels

    B. volcanic eruptions

    C. hydrolysis of water vapor by discharges of lightning in the atmosphere

    D. organisms that carry out photosynthesis

99- Among the choices below, which has the longest wavelength?

    A. orange wavelength visible light

    B. green wavelength visible light

    C. yellow wavelength visible light

    D. blue wavelength visible light

100-   Among the following, in a normal adult human the shortest bone(s) in the body is

    A. the femur

    B. the humerus

    C. The sternum

    D. The ribs

ADVANCED PRACTICE TEST: SCIENCE

1- Which of the following is a primary functional difference between smooth endoplasmic reticulum (SER) and rough endoplasmic reticulum (RER)?

    A. smooth endoplasmic reticulum does not participate in synthesis of products that are destined for external secretion.

    B. smooth endoplasmic reticulum does not participate in synthesis of proteins.

    C. Rough endoplasmic reticulum does not participate in synthesis of products that are destined for external secretion.

    D. rough endoplasmic reticulum does not participate in synthesis of proteins

2- Which of the following is a universal feature of all living cells?

    A. an external cell membrane

    B. an external cell wall

    C. a nucleus

    D. mitochondria

3- Which of the following terms would NOT be used to define the relative position of one body structure to another?

    A. caudal

    B. coronal

    C. ventral

    D. inferior

4- Which of the following identifies the type of intracellular filament that generates the whip-like motion of the flagellum of a human sperm cell?

    A. Thick filaments

    B. microfilaments

    C. microtubules

    D. intermediate filaments

5- Which of the following is NOT a characteristic of voluntary muscle tissue?

    A. synaptic muscle membrane interfaces with neurons

    B. high extracellular matrix volume

    C. high intracellular actin content

    D. electrically excitable cell membranes

6- Which of the following could be a nitrogenous base sequence of both a single codon and a single anticodon?

    A. ACG

    B. GCT

    C. UTC

    D. AGU

7- Which of the following is NOT a product molecule generated by a complete round of the Krebs (citric acid) cycle?

    A. CO_2

    B. acetyl CoA

    C. NADH

    D. $FADH_2$

8- Which of the following is an event that occurs during the successful maturation of a human primary follicle into a human secondary follicle?

    A. the corpus luteum degenerates

    B. a human sperm cell fertilizes the primary follicle

    C. a polar body is generated

    D. Increasing estrogen levels trigger a second luteinizing hormone (LH) peak.

9- Which of the following pairs of terms correctly completes the statement below?

In the human male reproductive system _____ cells produce _____.

    A. tunica albuginea; primary spermatids

    B. Sertoli; follicle stimulating hormone (FSH)

    C. spermatogonia; luteinizing hormone (LH)

    D. Leydig; testosterone

10- Which of the following pairs of terms correctly completes the statement below?

In humans, the ____ joint has a greater range of motion than the ____ joint.

    A. elbow; knee

    B. sacroiliac; atlanto axial

    C. elbow; shoulder

    D. knee; hip

11- Which of the following choices lists three organs that are all, to the greatest extent, derived from the same primary germ layer?

    A. heart, lung and kidney

    B. brain, heart and lung

    C. pancreas, liver, kidney

    D. lung, liver and pancreas

12- Which of the following is the primary function of pulmonary surfactant?

    A. prevention of rupture of alveoli during maximal inspiratory effort

    B. prevention of collapse of alveoli during exhalation

    C. increased solubility of oxygen in solution between alveoli and capillary endothelium

    D. decreased viscosity of bronchiolar luminal mucous secretions

13- Which of the following most likely does NOT increase during a maximal inspiratory effort compared to a normal (tidal) inspiratory effort?

    A. intrathoracic volume

    B. diffusion of CO_2 into alveolar airspaces

    C. pulmonary artery pressure

    D. diffusion of O_2 out of alveolar airspaces

14- Which of the following events occurs simultaneously with the end of systole?

    A. The aortic valve opens.

    B. The right ventricular pressure reaches a minimum value.

    C. The atrio-ventricular (A-V) node generates an electrical impulse.

    D. The mitral valve closes.

15- Among the choices below, within the cardiovascular system, which of the following in general has the lowest electrical conductivity?

    A. the atrioventricular septum

    B. intercalated discs

    C. Purkinje fibers

    D. The AV node

16- Which of the following is the most likely site for the origin of a blood clot that travels to and then lodges within the right main pulmonary artery?

    A. a peripheral vein located in the leg

    B. the aorta

    C. the left atrium

    D. a main pulmonary vein

17- Which of the following is by definition a lymphocyte lineage cell type?

    A. eosinophils

    B. plasma cells

    C. monocytes

    D. basophils

18- Dedicated or professional antigen presenting cells present antigens on their cell surfaces to T-cells in conjunction with which of the following types of cell membrane molecules?

    A. HLA class I antigens

    B. ABO glycoproteins

    C. Rh-factor proteins

    D. cadherin-class cell-adhesion molecules

19- Which of the following is NOT a cellular feature of enterocytes located in the small intestine?

    A. microvilli

    B. tight junctions

    C. desmosomes

    D. lacteals

20- Which of the following is most likely to lead to a suppression of the secretion of the hormone glucagon?

    A. high protein content of chyme in the stomach

    B. activation of the sympathetic nervous system

    C. a meal with high simple carbohydrate content

    D. the release of the hormone cholecystokinin (CCK)

21- Which of the following is a correct cause and effect sequence of events during the digestive process?

    A. CCK secretion→↑somatostatin secretion→↑pancreatic amylase secretion

    B. CCK secretion→↑bile secretion→↑fat emulsification

    C. secretin secretion→↑gastric mucous secretion→↑pepsin secretion

    D. secretin secretion→↑gastric HCL secretion→↑pepsin activation

22- Which of the following identifies the process responsible for the late hyperpolarization phase of an action potential?

A. sodium ion (Na+) diffusion into a neuron

B. sodium ion (Na+) diffusion out of a neuron

C. potassium ion (K+) diffusion into a neuron

D. potassium ion (K+) diffusion out of a neuron

23- Which of the following does not occur as a step in the physicochemical sequence that triggers sarcomere contraction within a myofibril?

    A. The release of norepinephrine (NE) into the neuron-myofibril gap of a neuromuscular junction

    B. The propagation of an electrical signal along a myofibril outer membrane into a T-tubule

    C. the release of CA++ ion from the sarcoplasmic reticulum of a myofibril

    D. the crosslink-binding of actin molecules and the "heads" of myosin molecules.

24- Which of the following pairs of cell types produce myelin sheaths?

    A. Schwann cells and oligodendroglia

    B. oligodendroglia and astrocytes

    C. astrocytes and Schwann cells

    D. microglia and neurons

25- Electrical signals to voluntary muscles most likely originate in which of the following locations in the central nervous system?

    A. the temporal lobes of the cerebral cortex

    B. the parietal lobes of the cerebral cortex

    C. the basal ganglia of the midbrain

    D. The cerebellum

26- Which of the following is most likely to directly result in the accumulation of lactic acid in muscle tissue?

    A. activation of the sympathetic nervous system

    B. depletion of glycogen stored in the liver

    C. inadequate amounts of O_2 delivered to muscle tissue

    D. inadequate levels of pyruvate within muscle tissue.

27- Which of the following is an effect of activation of the parasympathetic nervous system?

    A. increased activity of the sinoatrial node

    B. decreased activity of smooth muscle contractions in the wall of the digestive tract

    C. direct inhibition of deep tendon reflexes

    D. contraction of smooth muscle in the walls of arterioles in voluntary muscle tissue

28- On the outer membrane of a neuron, which of the following local regions would most likely contain the highest concentration of ligand-gated transmembrane ion channels?

A. axon terminals

B. junctional region of the axon and the main cell body (soma) of the neuron

C. dendrites

D. longitudinal mid-portion of the axon

29- Which of the following is the most precise anatomical location of the first stage of human spermatogenesis?

    A. the corpus spongiosum

    B. the seminiferous tubules

    C. the epididymis

    D. the seminal vesicles

30- Which of the following is the most precise location of the Bartholin's glands?

    A. immediately lateral to the labia majora

    B. medial to the labia majora and lateral to the labia minora

    C. medial to the labia minora and inferolateral to the vaginal introitus

    D. medial to the labia minora and superolateral to the urethral meatus

31- Which of the following correctly describes the course of a typical apocrine gland duct beginning at the duct's glandular origin and proceeding to the distal orifice of the duct?

    A. gland→hypodermis→basement membrane→dermis→shaft of hair follicle

    B. gland→dermis→basement membrane→epidermis→shaft of hair follicle

    C. a gland→hypodermis→basement membrane→dermis→external surface of the epidermis

    D. gland→dermis→basement membrane→epidermis→external surface of the epidermis

32- Which of the following describes the primary function of integumentary Langerhans cells?

    A. immune - antigen presentation

    B. somatosensory reception

    C. thermoregulation

    D structural adherence

33- Which of the following identifies the primary tissue type of the hypodermis and a primary function of the main cellular component of the hypodermis?

    A. epithelial; mechanical barrier

    B. epithelial energy storage

    C. connective; mechanical barrier

    D. connective; energy storage

34- Which of the following is NOT a hormone synthesized by the pituitary gland?

    A. prolactin

B. melatonin

C. oxytocin

D. adrenocorticotropic hormones (ACTH)

35- Which of the following hormones has rapid effects that are similar to effects associated with the activation of the sympathetic nervous system?

A. insulin

B. thyroid hormone (T3 and T4)

C. testosterone

D. aldosterone

36- Which of the following cell types initially secrets the majority of the hydroxyapatite component of lamellar bone?

A. osteoblasts

B. osteoclasts

C. osteocytes

D. fibroblasts

37- Which of the following is not a feature of or within trabecular (cancellous) bone?

A. red blood cell progenitor cells

B. white blood cell progenitor cells

C. haversian canals

D. adipocytes

38- Among the following, which choice identifies a join whose most general type is different from the other three?

A. frontal-sagittal joint

B. temporomandibular joint

C. sternomanubrial joint

D. sacroiliac joint

39- The initial filtration of blood by the kidney occurs at which of the following anatomical locations?

A. the renal pelvis

B. the adrenal cortex

C. the collecting ducts

D. the glomeruli

40- Which of the following is the kidney's response to exposure to antidiuretic hormone?

A. increased secretion of urea

B. decreased osmolality of extracellular fluid in the renal medulla

C. Increased renal tubule permeability to water

D. decreased secretion of glucose

41- Which of the following is the primary hormonal response of the central nervous system to an undesirably high plasma osmolarity?

    A. increased secretion of corticotropin releasing hormone

    B. decreased secretion of corticotropin releasing hormone

    C. increased secretion of antidiuretic hormone

    D. decreased secretion of antidiuretic hormone

42- Which of the following correctly completes the statement below?

    The effect of _____ on the kidney is the release of _____ by the kidney.

    A. an undesirably low plasma sodium ion concentration; renin

    B. an undesirably high plasma sodium ion concentration; renin

    C. an undesirably low plasma sodium ion concentration; aldosterone

    D. an undesirably high plasma sodium ion concentration; aldosterone

43- Under normal physiological circumstances, which of the following is completely reabsorbed by the kidney?

    A. glucose

    B. sodium

    C. bicarbonate ion

    D. urea

44- Which of the following is a physiological purpose of the sodium ion reabsorption-secretion cycle in the loop of Henle?

    A. sodium ion conservation

    B. potassium ion excretion

    C. concentration of urine

    D. acidification of urine

45- Which of the following is a DIRECT consequence of decreasing blood pressure on kidney function?

    A. decreased reabsorption of sodium ions

    B. decreased glomerular filtration rate (GFR)

    C. decreased secretion of renin

    D. increased secretion of aldosterone

46- Which of the following is a DIRECT physiological effect of angiotensin II?

    A. increased blood pressure

    B. increased renal medullary osmolality

    C. decreased renal tubule permeability to water

    D. redistribution of gastrointestinal blood flow

47- Which of the following are structurally required for the formation of a membrane attack complex (MAC)?

    A. perforins

    B. antigen specific antibodies

    C. platelet adhesion factors

    D. complement proteins

48- Which of the following does not participate in the immune response to viral infection?

    A. T-cells

    B. interferons

    C. chief cells

    D. plasma cells

49- Which of the following describes the mechanism of action of antivenom in snakebite victims?

    A. blockade of cell membrane molecular targets of snake venom toxin

    B. proteolytic destruction of the snake venom toxin molecules

    C. Non-enzymatic deamination of the snake venom toxin molecules

    D. deactivation of the snake venom toxin molecules by antigen-specific antibody binding

50- Which of the terms below correctly completes the following sentence?

The influenza vaccine provides _____ immunity to the influenza virus.

    A. active innate

    B. active humoral

    C. passive cellular

    D. passive innate

51- Which of the pairs of terms below correctly completes the following sentence?

Human T-cells originate from cells located in the_____ and reach maturity in the_____

    A. bone marrow; cortex of the spleen

    B. bone marrow; thymus

    C. thymus; cortex of the spleen

    D cortex of the spleen, thymus

52- Among the four cardinal signs of localized infection, which of the following is/are NOT the DIRECT result of increased vascular permeability?

    A. redness and swelling only

    B. redness and heat only

    C. swelling and pain only

D. pain and heat only

53- Which of the following is most clearly an autoimmune disease in humans?
  A. type 1 diabetes mellitus
  B. cystic fibrosis
  C. sickle cell anemia
  D. peptic ulcer disease

54- Which of the following identifies a direct causative sequence that results in the typical symptoms of seasonal pollen/mold allergies?
  A. antigen→mast cell release of peroxidase
  B. antigen→mast cell release of histamine
  C. antigen→Langerhans cell release of peroxidase
  D. antigen→Langerhans cell release of histamine

55- Which of the following diagrams the chemical reaction that results in the formation of a peptide bond between two amino acids, AA_1 and AA_2?
  A. $AA_1 + AA_2 \rightarrow AA_1\text{-}AA_2 + H_2O$
  B. $AA_1 + AA_2 \rightarrow AA_1\text{-}AA_2 + CO_2 + NH_3$
  C. $AA_1 + AA_2 \rightarrow AA_1\text{-}AA_2 + 2 \text{ glucose}$
  D. $AA_1 + AA_2 + NAD^+ \rightarrow AA_1\text{-}AA_2 + CO_2 + NADH$

56- Which of the following is an initial non-specific interaction between infectious bacteria and immune system cells that triggers activation of the innate immune system?
  A. immune sentinel cell membrane toll-like receptor binding to bacterial pathogen associated molecular patterns (PAMPs)
  B. antibody dependent cytotoxicity antibodies detected by natural killer cell membrane receptors
  C. cell membrane injury triggers conversion of cell membrane lipids to arachidonic acid
  D. down-regulation (removal) of class I MHC molecules from the surface of infected cells is recognized by T-helper cells

57- Which of the following correctly diagrams the synthesis of a triglyceride molecule?
  A. glycerol + 3 fatty acid molecules $\rightarrow$ triglyceride + 3 H_2O
  B. glycerol + 3 alkanes $\rightarrow$ triglyceride + 3 CO_2
  C. 3 glycerol + 3 fatty acid molecules $\rightarrow$ triglyceride + 3H_2O
  D. 3 glycerol + 3 alkanes $\rightarrow$ triglyceride + 3CO_2

58- Which of the following correctly diagrammatically summarizes glycogenesis in the liver?
  A. glucose molecules→ linear configuration glucose monomers in linear polymer chain molecules

B. glucose molecules→ cyclic configuration glucose monomers in linear polymer chain molecules

C. glucose molecules→ linear configuration glucose monomers in branching chain polymer molecules

D. glucose molecules→cyclic configuration glucose monomers in branching chain polymer molecules

59- Which of the following is a correct statement with regard to the molecular structure of human chromosomes?

   A. an individual chromatid always consists of one continuous single-strand form of a DNA molecule

   B. an individual chromatid always consists of one continuous s double-strand form of a DNA molecule

   C. an individual chromatid always consists of one continuous single-strand form of a DNA molecule

   D. an individual chromatid always consists of one continuous s double-strand form of a DNA molecule

60- Which of the following events could explain how a child could have three copies of chromosome 21 in all of his/her somatic cells?

   A. failure of separation of the chromosome 21 tetrad form during meiosis 1 division of gametogenesis

   B. failure of sister chromatid separation of chromosome 21 during a meiosis 2 division of gametogenesis

   C. failure of separation of the chromosome 21 tetrad form during the 2nd meiotic division of gametogenesis

   D. failure of sister chromatid separation of chromosome 21 during the first meiotic division of gametogenesis

61- Which of the following is NOT an error in the base pairing between two complementary strands of nucleic acid molecules?

   A. T-G

   B. G-A

   C. A-U

   D. C-T

62- Assume that there are a dominant and a recessive allele for each of two individual genes. The dominant gene alleles are P and Q and the recessive alleles are p and q. Which of the following are the predicted allelic inheritance frequencies of the two genes in offspring of parents where one parent is homozygous dominant for both genes and the other parent is homozygous recessive for both genes?

A. 100% PpQq

B. 50% PPQQ; 50% ppqq

C. 50% PPqq; 50% ppQQ

D. 25%PPQQ; 50%PpQq; 25% ppqq

63- The atoms of the elements argon and neon share which of the following characteristics?

A. a complete n=3 electron energy shell

B. positions located in the same period of the periodic table of the elements

C. filled valence octets

D. atomic diameter

64- The molecule CO_2 has which of the following characteristics?

A. approximately 109 degree bond angles.

B. two sigma bonds and two pi bonds

C. a molar weight of 24 atomic mass units (AMUs)

D. two lone-pairs of electrons

65- Which of the following crystalline solids contain ionic bonds with the least covalent character?

A. lithium fluoride (LiF)

B. magnesium chloride ($MgCl_2$)

C. potassium fluoride (KF)

D. calcium chloride ($CaCl_2$)

66- Among the choices below, which atoms have the highest 2nd ionization energy?

A. sodium

B. potassium

C. phosphorus

D. chlorine

67- Which of the following reversible reactions is catalyzed by the enzyme carbonic anhydrase?

A. $R_1\text{-COOH} + H_2N\text{-}R_2 \rightleftharpoons R_1CONHR_2 + H_2O$

B. acetyl CoA + $CO_2 \rightleftharpoons$ pyruvate

C. $CO_2 + H_2O \rightleftharpoons H_2CO_3$

D. $C_6H_{12}O_6 + 6O_2 \rightleftharpoons 6CO_2 + 6H_2O$

68- The function of which of the following peripheral nerves is most immediately essential to human life?

A. The vestibular nerves

B. the median nerves

C. the sciatic nerves

D. the phrenic nerves

69- Which of the following is a molecular compound that is directly produced by the normal catabolic pathway for the breakdown of hemoglobin?
   A. bilirubin
   B. uric acid
   C. urea
   D. bile

70- Which of the following pair of terms correctly completes the statement below?
   _____reversible reactions are always _____ reactions.
   A. exergonic forward, heat-producing forward
   B. endothermic forward, heat consuming reverse
   C. exothermic forward, spontaneous forward
   D endergonic forward, spontaneous reverse

71- Which of the following physical, phase-related properties of water is a deviation from the typical physical phase-related properties of other pure monomolecular substances?
   A. the ration of the substance's gas-phase density to its liquid-phase density is less than 1
   B. the ration of the substance's liquid-phase density to its solid-phase density is less than 1
   C. the ration of the substance's gas-phase density to its solid-phase density is less than 1
   D. the ration of the substance's plasma-phase density to its liquid-phase density is less than 1

72- Which of the following is NOT correct regarding the activation energy of a reversible reaction?
   A. The activation energy for the forward and reverse reactions is equal
   B. The rate of both the forward and reverse reactions increases when the activation energy decreases.
   C. The enthalpy for both the forward and reverse reactions is independent of the activation energy
   D. The entropy change for both the forward and reverse reactions is independent of the activation energy

73- Which of the following will tend to directly increase plasma pH levels?
   A. increased ventilation rate
   B. increased urinary excretion of bicarbonate ion
   C. increased anaerobic cellular respiration
   D. decreased tidal volume

74- In a sealed reaction vessel containing adequate volume to contain the volume of all liquid and gas components of a reaction, which of the following forward reactions of a reversible reaction will NOT be favored by increasing the volume of the reaction vessel? Note: (g) = gas phase, (l) = liquid phase and (s) = solid phase

A. $A(g) + B(g) \rightleftharpoons C(g) + 2\,D(g)$

B. $A(g) + 4\,B(s) \rightleftharpoons C(g) + D(g)$

C. $2\,A(g) + 2\,B(g) \rightleftharpoons 4\,C(s) + D(g)$

D. $3\,A(l) + 2\,B(g) \rightleftharpoons 2\,C(g) + D(g)$

75- Which of the following changes in the temperature of H_2O at standard temperature and pressure requires the greatest input of heat energy?

    A. -3 Celsius to 0 Celsius

    B. -2 Celsius to 1 Celsius

    C. 97 Celsius to 100 Celsius

    D. 102 Celsius to 105 Celsius

76- In a sealed container filled only with gas molecules, where the container volume = V, the gas temperature = T and the gas pressure = P, which of the following expressions is directly proportional to the number of moles of gas in the container?

    A. $(P)(V)/T$

    B. $(P)(T)/V$

    C. $(T)(V)/P$

    D. $V/(T)(P)$

77- The addition of 100 ml of pure liquid water will lower the pH of a 1 liter volume of which of the following solutions by the greatest amount?

    A. a solution with a pH = 8

    B. a solution with a pH = 7

    C. a solution with a pH = 6

    D. a solution with a pH = 5

78- Which of the following statements is true regarding the reaction of 1 liter of a 0.1 molar strong acid (HA) aqueous solution with a one liter of a 0.1 molar weak base (BOH) aqueous solution? Note: In this question the conjugate base A- and conjugate acid B+ do not form a salt (AB) that precipitates out of solution.

    A. the resultant solution will have a pH of 7

    B. the resultant solution will have a pH that is greater than 7

    C. the concentration of HA will be greater than the concentration of BOH in the resultant solution.

    D. The combined concentration of the conjugate base A- and conjugate acid B+ in the resultant solution will be greater than the combined concentration of conjugate acid B+ and OH- in the resultant solution

79- Which of the following MUST be true regarding two sealed samples of different monomolecular gases that have the same temperature?

A. The gas molecules in both samples have the same molecular mass

B. The gas molecules in both samples have the same average velocity

C. The gas molecules in both samples have the same average ratio of mass to velocity

D. The gas molecules in both samples have the same average kinetic energy

80- Which of the following choices represents as sample of a substance that consists of 6.022×10^{23} molecules?

    A. 1 liter of H_2O gas at standard pressure and temperature

    B. 20 liters of N_2 gas at standard pressure and temperature

    C. 18 grams of liquid H_2O

    D. 8 grams of liquid CH_4

81- Which of the following is the pressure at the bottom of the inside of a sealed cylindrical vessel with an internal cross-sectional area of $1 \ m^2$ that is completely filled by a liquid substance with a mass of 1 kg?

    A. 9.8 pressure units

    B. $9.8 / \pi^2$ pressure units

    C. $(4.9) \pi$ pressure units

    D. $(4.9) \pi^2$ pressure units

82- Which of the following is velocity (v) of a 100 kilogram (kg) object that has that has a kinetic energy (KE) of 500 joules (J)?

    A. 1 m/s

    B. 2 m/s

    C. 5 m/s

    D. 10 m/s

83- Which of the following is the density of a solid sphere with a radius of 1 meter (m) and a mass of 4 kg?

    A. (4)(9.8) density units

    B. $3 / \pi$ density units

    C. $9.8 \ \pi^3$ density units

    D. 4 density units

84- Which of the following is most nearly the sum of the masses of one proton, one neutron and one electron?

    A. 1×10^{-3} amu

    B. 2 amu

    C. 3 amu

    D. 1×10^3 amu

85- Which of the following pairs of atoms have the largest ratio of nuclear charge?
   A. helium to hydrogen
   B. nitrogen to carbon
   C. chlorine to magnesium
   D. krypton to potassium

86- In humans, the complete absence of which of the following hormones would represent the most immediate threat to life without medical treatment?
   A. oxytocin
   B. cortisol
   C. insulin
   D. melatonin

87- Which of the following has the lowest percentage content of collagen?
   A. compact bone
   B. ligaments
   C. tendons
   D. cartilage

88- In Humans, which of the following has the highest percentage content of protein arranged in helical structures?
   A. testosterone
   B. keratin
   C. hemoglobin
   D. DNA

89- Which of the following INCORRECTLY identifies one or both functional groups shown in the answer choices below? Note: "R" represents a hydrocarbon group. Note: The functional groups in some cases could instead be bonded to groups other than R groups - the indicated carbons of the functional groups all will bond to carbons of hydrocarbon R groups as represented in the answer choices.
   A. $CH_4 \rightarrow$ alkane; $R\text{-}CH_2OH \rightarrow$ alcohol
   B. $R\text{-}COOH \rightarrow$ carboxylic acid; $R\text{-}CO\text{-}R \rightarrow$ ketone
   C. $R\text{-}NH_2 \rightarrow$ amine; $R\text{-}CH=CH2 \rightarrow$ alkene
   D. $R\text{-}O\text{-}R \rightarrow$ ether; $R\text{-}COO\text{-}R \rightarrow$ aldehyde

90- If the equilibrium constant (K_{eq}) for a reversible chemical reaction is $K_{eq}=1$, which of the following is a correct equation for the reaction if at equilibrium the concentrations of all of the participants in the reaction are equal?
   A. $A + B \leftrightharpoons C$
   B. $A + B \leftrightharpoons 2C$

C. $2A + 2B \leftrightharpoons C$

D. $2A + 2B \leftrightharpoons 2C$

91- Which of the following conditions would be MOST likely to increase to risk for osteoporosis?
   A. high testosterone levels in males
   B. vitamin E deficiency
   C. subnormal ovarian function
   D. hyperactive adrenal medullary gland function

92- Which of the following is an INCORRECT pairing of a disease and a major risk factor for the disease?
   A. myocardial infarction → high HDL cholesterol levels
   B. stroke → high blood pressure
   C. malignant melanoma → sunlight exposure
   D. bacterial pneumonia → surgical removal of the spleen (splenectomy)

93- Which of the following is the dominant/recessive type and chromosomal location of the gene that is responsible for the most common form of inherited color-blindness?
   A. chromosome 21, dominant
   B. chromosome 21, recessive
   C. X chromosome, dominant
   D. X chromosome, recessive

94- Which of the following vitamin deficiencies can cause anemia that does not improve with the administration of daily oral iron supplementation?
   A. vitamin B-12 deficiency
   B. vitamin C deficiency
   C. vitamin D deficiency
   D. vitamin K deficiency

95- Which of the following the nucleic acid type of the human immunodeficiency virus (HIV) and the cell target of the HIV virus in the human immune system?
   A. DNA virus; T-helper cells (CD4 cells)
   B. DNA virus; cytotoxic T-cells (CD8 cells)
   C. RNA virus; T-helper cells (CD4 cells)
   D. RNA virus; cytotoxic T-cells (CD8 cells)

96- Which of the following correctly completes the statement below?
   The carotid and aortic bodies measure the _____ and relay this information to the_____.
   A. partial pressure of arterial O_2: pons and medulla oblongata
   B. partial pressure of arterial CO_2: pons and medulla oblongata

C. partial pressure of arterial O_2: hypothalamus

D. partial pressure of arterial O_2: hypothalamus

97- Which of the following hormones regulates overall energy metabolism and modulates the body's immune system responses?

    A. thyroid hormone (T3 and T4)

    B. cortisol

    C. calcitonin

    D. parathyroid hormone (PTH)

98- Which of the following separate genetic traits are least likely to follow the mendelian law of independent assortment?

    A. traits resulting from genes located on the sex chromosomes (X and Y chromosomes)

    B. traits resulting from genes located on different autosomal chromosome pairs

    C. traits resulting from genes located at either terminal pole of the same chromosome

    D. traits resulting from genes located adjacent to each other on the same chromosome

99- Which of the following vessels normally experiences the highest levels of free amino acids in the bloodstream?

    A. the splenic vein

    B. the hepatic portal vein

    C. the renal glomerular capillaries

    D. the thoracic duct.

100- The term mycosis refers to which of the following?

    A. excessive myoglobin levels in the bloodstream

    B. a fungal infection

    C. an inherited abnormality of myosin proteins in muscle cells

    D. nearsightedness

ADVANCED PRACTICE TEST: MATHEMATICS

1 – Change to an improper fraction. 2 1/3

    A. 5/3

    B. 3/7

    C. 7/3

    D. 8/3

2 – Which of the following is equivalent to 60% of 90?

    A. 0.6 x 90

    B. 90 ÷ 0.6

    C. 3/5

D. 2/3

3 – Convert the improper fraction $^{17}/_6$ to a mixed number.
   A. $1\,^7/_6$
   B. $2\,^5/_6$
   C. $^6/_{17}$
   D. $2\,^7/_6$

4 – The decimal value of 7/11 is _____?
   A. 1.57
   B. 0.70
   C. 0.6363…
   D. 0.77

5 – The decimal value of 5/8 is _____?
   A. 0.625
   B. 0.650
   C. 0.635
   D. 0.580

6 – The fractional value of 0.5625 is _____?
   A. 7/15
   B. 11/23
   C. 5/8
   D. 9/16

7 – The fractional value of 0.3125 is _____?
   A. 5/16
   B. 4/24
   C. 6/19
   D. 9/25

8 – What is the value of this expression if $a = 10$ and $b = -4$:
$$\sqrt{b^2 - 2 \bullet a}$$
   A. 6
   B. 7
   C. 8
   D. 9

9 – What is the greatest common factor of 48 and 64?
   A. 4
   B. 8
   C. 16

D. 32

10 – Solve for *x*: $X = \frac{3}{4} \bullet \frac{7}{8}$
- A. 7/8
- B. 9/8
- C. 10/12
- D. 21/32

11 – Find the value of $a^2 + 6b$ when $a = 3$ and $b = 0.5$.
- A. 12
- B. 6
- C. 9
- D. 15

12 – What is the least common multiple of 8 and 10?
- A. 80
- B. 40
- C. 18
- D. 72

13 – What is the sum of 1/3 and 3/8?
- A. 3/24
- B. 4/11
- C. 17/24
- D. 15/16

14 – Solve this equation: $-9 \bullet -9 =$
- A. 18
- B. 0
- C. 81
- D. –81

15 – Which of the following is between 2/3 and 3/4?
- A. 3/5
- B. 4/5
- C. 7/10
- D. 5/8

16 – Which digit is in the thousandths place in the number: 1,234.567
- A. 1
- B. 2

C. 6

D. 7

17 – Which of these numbers is largest?

    A. 5/8

    B. 3/5

    C. 2/3

    D. 0.72

18 – Which of these numbers is largest?

    A. −345

    B. 42

    C. −17

    D. 3^4

19 – Find 4 numbers between 4.857 and 4.858

    A. 4.8573, 4.85735, 4.85787, 4.8598

    B. 4.857, 4.8573, 4.8578, 4.8579,

    C. 4.8571, 4.8573, 4.8578, 4.8579

    D. 4.8572, 4.8537, 4.8578, 4.8579

20 – Which number is between 4 and 5?

    A. 11/3

    B. 21/4

    C. 31/6

    D. 23/5

21 – Which number is not between 7 and 9?

    A. 34/5

    B. 29/4

    C. 49/6

    D. 25/3

22 – If $\dfrac{4}{9}x - 3 = 1$, what is the value of x?

    A. 9

    B. 8

    C. 7

    D. −4½

23 – What value of q is a solution to this equation: $130 = q(-13)$

    A. 10

B. –10

C. 1

D. 10^2

24 – Solve this equation: x = –12 ÷ –3

    A. $x = -4$

    B. $x = -15$

    C. $x = 9$

    D. $x = 4$

25 – Solve for *r* in the equation $p = 2r + 3$

    A. r = 2p – 3

    B. r = p + 6

    C. r = (p - 3) / 2

    D. r = p – 3/2

26 – Solve this equation: $x = 8 - (-3)$

    A. $x = 5$

    B. $x = -5$

    C. $x = 11$

    D. $x = -11$

27 – Evaluate the expression $7x^2 + 9x - 18$ for x = 7

    A. 516

    B. 424

    C. 388

    D. 255

28 – Evaluate the expression $x^2 + 7x - 18$ for x = 5

    A. 56

    B. 42

    C. 38

    D. 25

29 – Evaluate the expression $7x^2 + 63x$ for x = 27

    A. 5603

    B. 4278

    C. 6804

    D. 6525

30 – Sam worked 40 hours at *d* dollars per hour and received a bonus of $50. His total earnings were $530. What was his hourly wage?

    A. $18

B. $16

C. $14

D. $12

31 – The variable X is a positive integer. Dividing X by a positive number less than 1 will yield

A. a number greater than X

B. a number less than X

C. a negative number

D. an irrational number

32 – Amanda makes $14 an hour as a bank teller and Oscar makes $24 dollars an hour as an auto mechanic. Both work eight hours a day, five days a week. Which of these equations can be used to calculate how much they make together in a five-day week?

A. $(14 + 24) \cdot 8 \cdot 5$

B. $14 \cdot 24 \cdot 8 \cdot 5$

C. $(14 + 24) (8 + 5)$

D. $14 + 24 \cdot 8 \cdot 5$

33 – Seven added to four-fifths of a number equals fifteen. What is the number?

A. 10

B. 15

C. 20

D. 25

34 – If the sum of two numbers is 360 and their ratio is 7:3, what is the smaller number?

A. 72

B. 105

C. 98

D. 108

35 – Jean buys a textbook, a flash drive, a printer cartridge, and a ream of paper. The flash drive costs three times as much as the ream of paper. The textbook costs three times as much as the flash drive. The printer cartridge costs twice as much as the textbook. The ream of paper costs $10. How much does Jean spend altogether?

A. $250

B. $480

C. $310

D. $180

36 – The area of a triangle equals one-half the base times the height. Which of the following is the correct way to calculate the area of a triangle that has a base of 6 and a height of 9?

    A. (6 + 9)/2
    B. ½(6 + 9)
    C. 2(6 x 9)
    D. $\dfrac{(6)(9)}{2}$

37 – Calculate the value of this expression: $2 + 6 \cdot 3 \cdot (3 \cdot 4)^2 + 1$

    A. 2,595
    B. 5,185
    C. 3,456
    D. 6,464

38 – A rectangle of length and width 3x and x has an area of $3x^2$. Write the area polynomial when the length is increased by 5 units and the width is decreased by 3 units. (3x+5) (x-3)

    A. $3x^2 +14x - 15$
    B. $3x^2 - 4x - 15$
    C. $3x^2 - 5x + 15$
    D. $3x^2 + 4x - 15$

39 – A triangle of base and height 4x and 7x has an area of $14x^2$, which is equal ½ times the base times the height. Write the area polynomial when the base is increased by 2 units and the height is increased by 3 units. ½ (4x+2)(7x+3)

    A. $14x^2 +14x +6$
    B. $14x^2 +14x +3$
    C. $14x^2 +13x + 3$
    D. $14x^2 + 28x +3$

40 – Momentum is defined as the product of mass times velocity. If your 1,250 kg car is travelling at 55 km/hr, what is the value of the momentum?

    A. 68,750 kg m/s
    B. 19,098 kg m/s
    C. 9,549 kg m/s
    D. 145,882 kg m/s

41 – In her retirement accounts, Janet has invested $40,000 in stocks and $65,000 in bonds. If she wants to rebalance her accounts so that 70% of her investments are in stocks, how much will she have to move?

    A. $33,500
    B. $35,000
    C. $37,500
    D. $40,000

42 – Brian pays 15% of his gross salary in taxes. If he pays $7,800 in taxes, what is his gross salary?

    A. $52,000

    B. $48,000

    C. $49,000

    D. $56,000

43 – In a high school French class, 45% of the students are sophomores, and there are 9 sophomores in the class. How many students are there in the class?

    A. 16

    B. 18

    C. 20

    D. 22

44 – Marisol's score on a standardized test was ranked in the 78th percentile. If 660 students took the test, approximately how many students scored lower than Marisol?

    A. 582

    B. 515

    C. 612

    D. 486

45 – The population of Mariposa County in 2015 was 90% of its population in 2010. The population in 2010 was 145,000. What was the population in 2010?

    A. 160,000

    B. 142,000

    C. 120,500

    D. 130,500

46 – Alicia must have a score of 75% to pass a test of 80 questions. What is the greatest number of question she can miss and still pass the test?

    A. 20

    B. 25

    C. 60

    D. 15

47 – A cell phone on sale at 30% off costs $210. What was the original price of the phone?

    A. $240

    B. $273

    C. $300

    D. $320

48 – In the graduating class at Emerson High School, 52% of the students are girls and 48% are boys. There are 350 students in the class. Among the girls, 98 plan to go to college. How many girls do not plan to go to college?

  A. 84
  B. 48
  C. 66
  D. 72

49 – The number of students enrolled at Two Rivers Community College increased from 3,450 in 2010 to 3,864 in 2015. What was the percent increase?

  A. 9%
  B. 17%
  C. 12%
  D. 6%

50 – Produce is usually priced to the nearest pound. A scale for weighing produce has numerical values for pounds and ounces. Which of the following weights would you expect to be priced for 15 pounds?

  A. 15 pounds 14 ounces
  B. 15 pounds 10 ounces
  C. 14 pounds 4 ounces
  D. 14 pounds 14 ounces

51 – Which number is rounded to the nearest ten-thousandth?

  A. 7,510,000
  B. 7,515,000
  C. 7,514,635.8239
  D. 7,514,635.824

52 – Measuring devices determine the precision of our scientific measurements. A graduated cylinder is used that has a maximum of 10 cc's but has ten increments in between each whole number of cc's. Which answer is a correct representation of a volume measurement with this cylinder?

  A. 7 cc's
  B. 7.1 cc's
  C. 7.15 cc's
  D. 7.514 cc's

53 – If a man can unload about 50 pounds in a time of 15 minutes, estimate the time and labor force to unload 2.5 tons of 50 pound blocks from a truck working 8 hours per day.

  A. 1 man for 10 days

B. 2 men for 1 day

C. 4 men for 1 day

D. 5 men for 5 days

54 – In rush hour, you can usually commute 18 miles to work in 45 minutes. If you believe that you can travel an average of 5 miles per hour faster in the early morning, how much time would you estimate for the early commute to work?

    A. 50 minutes

    B. 40 minutes

    C. 30 minutes

    D. 20 minutes

55 – You are taking a test and you are allowed to work a class period of 45 minutes. 20 problems are multiple choice and 30 of the problems are true / false. If they have equal value, how much time would you estimate for each type of problem if you believe you are twice as fast at multiple choice problems?

    A. 90 seconds per m/c; 45 seconds per t/f

    B. 60 seconds per m/c; 30 seconds per t/f

    C. 70 seconds per m/c; 35 seconds per t/f

    D. 80 seconds per m/c; 40 seconds per t/f

56 – Your interview is scheduled for 8:00 in the morning and you need to allow 20 minutes for your trip to the interview. You oversleep and leave 10 minutes late. How fast will you travel to get there on time?

    A. half as fast

    B. twice as fast

    C. three times as fast

    D. four times as fast

57 – A square meter is a square with sides that are one meter in length. If a meter is 1000 millimeters, how many square millimeters are in a square meter.

    A. 100

    B. 1000

    C. 10,000

    D. 1,000,000

58 – In four years, Tom will be twice as old as Serena was three years ago. Tom is three years younger than Serena. How old are Tom and Serena?

    A. Serena is 28, Tom is 25

    B. Serena is 7, Tom is 4

    C. Serena is 18, Tom is 15

D. Serena is 21, Tom is 18

59 – Amy drives her car until the gas gauge is down to 1/8 full. Then she fills the tank by adding 14 gallons. What is the capacity of the gas tank?

    A. 16 gallons

    B. 18 gallons

    C. 20 gallons

    D. 22 gallons

60 – Two rectangles are proportional; that is, the ratio of length to width is the same for both rectangles. The smaller rectangle has a length of 8 inches and a width of 3 inches. The large rectangle has a length of 12 inches. What is the width of the larger rectangle?

    A. 4 inches

    B. 4.5 inches

    C. 6 inches

    D. 8.5inches

61 – The perimeter of a rectangle is 24 inches, and the ratio of the length to the width is 2:1. What is the area of the rectangle?

    A. 60 square inches

    B. 18 square inches

    C. 32 square inches

    D. 48 square inches

62 – The tree near your house casts a shadow of 27 feet. At the same time of day, your house which is 40 feet tall at the peak of the roof casts a shadow of 68 feet. The tree height must be _____.

    A. 100 feet tall

    B. 16 feet tall

    C. 45 feet tall

    D. 20 feet tall

63 – Five students volunteered to paint a room in the community center. If the painters estimated they would finish the job with 2 ½ man-days, how long should it take the students?

    A. Two days

    B. One day

    C. Half a day

    D. One quarter of a day

64 – Your car can maintain 23 miles per gallon on the freeway. If you are travelling to Oklahoma City, which is about 500 miles north, how much gasoline will be required for the trip?

A. 37 gallons

B. 53 gallons

C. 105 gallons

D. 22 gallons

65 – On your trip, you find that it takes you 8.5 hours to get to Oklahoma City which is 500 miles north. How much more time should it take to get to Wichita, Kansas (640 miles total)

A. 7 hours

B. 5 hours

C. 11 hours

D. 2.5 hours

66 – Eight machines can produce 96 parts per minute. How many parts could 12 identical machines produce in 3 minutes?

A. 144

B. 288

C. 256

D. 432

67 – At Pleasantville College, the ratio of female to male students is exactly 5 to 4. Which of the following could be the number of students at the college?

A. 8,200

B. 2,955

C. 3,500

D. 3,105

68 – When you add two numbers, the sum is 480. The ratio of the two numbers is 5:1, what is the smaller number?

A. 60

B. 70

C. 72

D. 80

69 – Four friends plan to share the cost of a retirement gift equally. If one person drops out of the arrangement, the cost per person for the other three would increase by $12. What is the cost of the gift?

A. $144

B. $136

C. $180

D. $152

70 – It took Charles four days to write a history paper. He wrote 5 pages on the first day, 4 pages on the second day, and 8 pages on the third day. If Charles wrote an average of 7 pages per day, how many pages did he write on the fourth day?

    A. 11

    B. 8

    C. 12

    D. 9

71 – How much weight must you lose each week if you are determined to lose 63 pounds in 6 months?

    A. 0.4 lbs. per week

    B. 2.4 lbs. per week

    C. 1.4 lbs. per week

    D. 0.64 lbs. per week

72 – How much money must you save each week if you are determined to have $375 in the next 7 months?

    A. $12.38 per week

    B. $11.50 per week

    C. $13.75 per week

    D. $7. 75 per week

73 – If you think that you can save $450 out of your monthly pay check, how long will it take for you to save $3995 for your car down payment?

    A. 8 months

    B. 10 months

    C. 9 weeks

    D. 9 months

74 – You have read that your car is losing value at a rate of $55 per month. You are asking $1790 and a potential buyer has offered you $1450. How many months will it take before you can accept that offer?

    A. 8 months

    B. 6 months

    C. 15 weeks

    D. 4 months

75 – The product of two numbers is 6 more than the sum of the two numbers. Which of these equations describes this relationship?

    A. $X \bullet Y + 6 = X + Y$

    B. $X \bullet Y = X + Y + 6$

    C. $X + Y = X + Y - 6$

    D. $X \bullet Y = X + Y - 6$

76 – There are 3 more men than women on the board of directors of the Big Box Retail Company. There are 13 members of the board. How many are women?

    A. 3

    B. 4

    C. 5

    D. 6

77 – The average of 25, 35, and 120 is 10 more than the average of 40, 45, and which value?

    A. 60

    B. 65

    C. 70

    D. 76

78 – What is the smallest positive integer that is evenly divisible by 5 and 7 and leaves a remainder of 4 when divided by 6?

    A. 35

    B. 70

    C. 105

    D. 140

79 – The ratio of female to male nurses in a hospital is 9:1. If there are 144 female nurses, how many male nurses are there?

    A. 12

    B. 14

    C. 16

    D. 18

80 – Of the patients admitted to an ER over a one-week period, 14 had heart attacks, 15 had workplace injuries, 24 were injured in auto accidents, 12 had respiratory problems, 21 were injured in their homes, and 34 had other medical problems. What percent of patients had respiratory problems?

    A. 10%

    B. 12%

    C. 15%

    D. 18%

81 – Alan commutes 18 miles to work. Bob's commute is 4 miles shorter. Ted's commute is 6 miles shorter than Bob's. Rebecca's commute is shorter than Alan's but longer than Bob's. Which of the following could be the length of Rebecca's commute?

    A. 12 miles

    B. 14 miles

    C. 15 miles

    D. 18 miles

82 – At a lunch cart there are 2 orders of diet soda for every 5 orders of regular soda. If the owner of the lunch cart sells 112 sodas a day, how many are diet and how many are regular?

    A. 28 diet, 84 regular

    B. 32 diet, 80 regular

    C. 34 diet, 82 regular

    D. 36 diet, 84 regular

83 – The three teams with the best records in the division are the Bulldogs, the Rangers, and the Statesmen. The Bulldogs have won nine games and lost three. The Rangers have won ten games and lost two. The Statesmen have also won ten games and lost two. Each team has one game left before the playoffs. The Bulldogs will be playing the Black Sox, and the Rangers will be playing the Statesmen. The team with the best record will win a spot in the playoffs. Which of the following statements is true?

    A. The Statesmen will definitely be in the playoffs.

    B. The Bulldogs will definitely not be in the playoffs.

    C. The Rangers will definitely not be in the playoffs.

    D. The Statesmen will definitely not be in the playoffs.

84 – At Pleasantville College, the ratio of female to male students is exactly 5 to 4. Which of the following could be the number of students at the college?

    A. 8,200

    B. 2,955

    C. 3,500

    D. 3,105

85 – Which equation is shown on this graph?

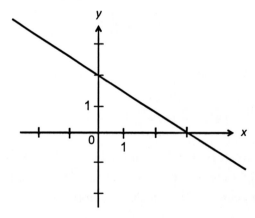

    A. $y = 2x + 1$

B. y = –2/3x + 2
C. y = –3x + 1
D. y = 3x + 2

86 – If the y-intercept of the line on this graph was reduced by 1, what would be the slope of the line?

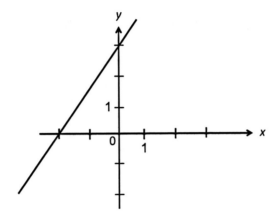

A. –1
B. –2
C. 2
D. 1

87 – Each figure (ß) is valued at $450 . Which of the following is valued closest to $6,500?
A. ß/2
B. ß ß ß ß ß ß ß ß ß
C. ß ß ß ß ß ß ß ß ß ß ß ß ß ß ß ß/2
D. ß ß ß ß ß

88 – Kevin has his glucose levels checked monthly. These are the results:

January	February	March	April	May	June	July
98	102	88	86	110	92	90

In which month was his glucose level equal to the median level for these seven months?
A. January
B. March
C. April
D. June

89 – The average weight of five friends (Al, Bob, Carl, Dave, and Ed) is 180 pounds. Al weighs 202 pounds, Bob weighs 166 pounds, Carl weighs 190 pounds, and Dave weighs 192 pounds. How much does Ed weigh?

    A. 180 pounds

    B. 172 pounds

    C. 186 pounds

    D. 150 pounds

90 – What is the mode in this set of numbers: 4, 5, 4, 8, 10, 4, 6, 7

    A. 6

    B. 4

    C. 8

    D. 7

91 – Find the median in this series of numbers: 80, 78, 73, 69, 100.

    A. 69

    B. 73

    C. 78

    D. 80

92 – Your scholarship requires a 93% average in your Medical Terminology class. Your grades so far are in this class are 88, 90, 95, 92, 87, 89, 90, 95. With two grades left, what average do you need to have for those two grades to maintain your scholarship?

    A. 97

    B. 99

    C. 101

    D. 102

93 – The x/y values for your data look like the following table:

X	3	5	7	9	11	13	15	17
Y	22	19	16	13	10	7	4	1

The y-intercept is defined as the y value when x = 0. The y-intercept for the data table in this problem is:

    A. 8

    B. 19.7

    C. 25

    D. 26.5

94 – Which of the following represents the relationship between x and y in this table?

x	y
0	7
3	13
5	17
7	21
8	23

A. $y = x + 7$
B. $y = 4x + 1$
C. $y = 2x + 10$
D. $y = 2x + 7$

95 – If a patient's weight is recorded each day for a two-week period, a graph of this data would most likely be presented with:
A. y axis with height and x axis with date
B. y axis with weight and x axis with time
C. y axis with dates and x axis with weight
D. y axis with weight and x axis with date

96 – The weather channel says that the temperature will be 45 degrees on Monday and increasing 5 degrees each day for the Tuesday through Sunday. With this description, which best describes the dependent and independent variables?
A. The day depends on the temperature
B. Days are the independent variable
C. Temperature is the independent variable
D. There is no correlation between day and temperature

97 – A critical care patient has lost 15 pounds during the hospital stay. In terms of the mathematical model of this data, it is labelled as a(n) _____
A. positive covariation
B. negative covariation
C. independent variable covariation
D. random covariation

98 – A rectangle has a length of 8 and a width of 6. What would be the side of a square with the same perimeter?
A. 5
B. 6

C. 7

D. 8

99 – Which of the following can be the lengths of the sides of a triangle?

    A. 1,2,4

    B. 2,4,8

    C. 2,3,4

    D. 4,5,9

100 – A square 8 inches on a side is cut into smaller squares 1 inch on a side. How many of the smaller squares can be made?

    A. 8

    B. 16

    C. 24

    D. 64

101 – What is the perimeter of this figure?

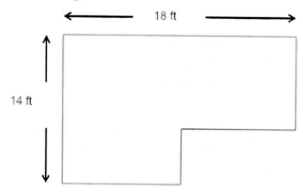

    A. 64 ft.

    B. 72 ft.

    C. 84 ft.

    D. 96 ft.

102 – If the radius of the circle in this diagram is 4 inches, what is the perimeter of the square?

    A. 24 inches

    B. 32 inches

C. 64 inches

D. 96 inches

103 – A rectangle's length is three times its width. The area of the rectangle is 48 square feet. How long are the sides?

    A. length = 12, width = 4

    B. length = 15, width = 5

    C. length = 18, width = 6

    D. length = 24, width = 8

104 – Danvers is 8 miles due south of Carson and 6 miles due west of Baines. If a driver could drive in a straight line from Carson to Baines, how long would the trip be?

    A. 8 miles

    B. 10 miles

    C. 12 miles

    D. 14 miles

105 – Carmen has a box that is 18 inches long, 12 inches wide, and 14 inches high. What is the volume of the box?

    A. 44 cubic inches

    B. 3,024 cubic inches

    C. 216 cubic inches

    D. 168 cubic inches

106 – Which of the following is equal to 0.0065?

    A. 6.5×10^{-2}

    B. 6.5×10^{-3}

    C. 6.5×10^{-4}

    D. 6.5×10^{-5}

107 – If one inch is equal to 25.4 millimeters, how many millimeters are in a 20 foot long steel beam

    A. 6506

    B. 6906

    C. 6609

    D. 6096

108 – Medical doses are often measured in cubic centimeters or cc's. A rectangular volume that has a volume of 100 cc's and a square base with 4 inches on each side must must be how tall?

    A. 9.7 millimeters

    B. 6.5 centimeters

    C. 103 centimeters

    D. 10.3 millimeters

109 – Small motorcycles often have a displacement of 100 cc's or less. This represents _____
    cubic inches?
    A. 61 cubic inches
    B. 15.5 cubic inches
    C. 6.1 cubic inches
    D. 39.4 cubic inches

110 – A medical dose is listed as 25 milligrams for each capsule. If there are thirty capsules in the
    bottle. How many kilograms of the drug are in the bottle?
    A. 0.00075 kg
    B. 750 g
    C. 250 g
    D. 0.00050 kg

INTERMEDIATE PRACTICE TEST: ENGLISH

1. Which of the following choices best completes this sentence?
    When asked if the sleeping pill had _____ him at all, the man replied
    that it had had no _____; nonetheless, he realized that he
    _____not attempt to drive his car that evening.
    A. affected; effect; ought
    B. affected; effect; aught
    C. effected; affect; ought
    D. effected; affect; aught

2. Which sentence makes best use of grammatical conventions for clarity and concision?
    A. Hiking along the trail, the birds chirped loudly and interrupted our attempt at a peaceful
       nature walk.
    B. The birds chirped loudly, attempting to hike along the nature trail we were interrupted.
    C. Hiking along the trail, we were assailed by the chirping of birds, which made our nature
       walk hardly the peaceful exercise we had wanted.
    D. Along the nature trail, our walk was interrupted by loudly chirping birds in our attempt
       at a nature trail.

3. Which word from the following sentence is an adjective?
    A really serious modern-day challenge is finding a way to consume real food in a world of overly
    processed food products.
    A. really
    B. challenge
    C. consume
    D. processed

4. To improve sentence fluency, how could you state the information below in a single sentence? My daughter was in a dance recital. I attended it with my husband. She received an award. We were very proud.
    A. My daughter, who was in a dance recital, received an award, which made my husband and I, who were in attendance, very proud.
    B. My husband and I attended my daughter's dance recital and were very proud when she received an award.
    C. Attending our daughter's dance recital, my husband and I were very proud to see her receive an award.
    D. Dancing in a recital, my daughter received an award which my husband and I, who were there, very proud.

5. Which sentence is punctuated correctly?
    A. Since the concert ended very late I fell asleep in the backseat during the car ride home.
    B. Since the concert ended very late: I fell asleep in the backseat during the car ride home.
    C. Since the concert ended very late; I fell asleep in the backseat during the car ride home.
    D. Since the concert ended very late, I fell asleep in the backseat during the car ride home.

6. Which of the choices below best completes the following sentence?
   Negotiations with the enemy are never fun, but during times of war
   _____ a necessary evil.
    A. its
    B. it's
    C. their
    D. they're

7. Which of the verbs below best completes the following sentence?
   The a cappela group _____ looking forward to performing for the entire student body at the graduation ceremony.
    A. is
    B. are
    C. was
    D. be

8. What kind of sentence is this?
   I can't believe her luck!
    A. Declarative
    B. Imperative
    C. Exclamatory
    D. Interrogative

9. Identify the error in this sentence:
   Irregardless of the expense, it is absolutely imperative that all drivers have liability insurance to cover any personal injury that may be suffered during a motor vehicle accident.
    A. Irregardless
    B. Imperative
    C. Liability
    D. Suffered

10. Which of the following sentences is grammatically correct?
    A. Between you and me, I brang back less books from my dorm room than I needed to study for my exams.
    B. Between you and I, I brought back less books from my dorm room then I needed to study for my exams.
    C. Between you and me, I brought back fewer books from my dorm room than I needed to study for my exam.
    D. Between you and me, I brought back fewer books from my dorm room then I needed to study for my exams.

11. Choose from the answers to complete this sentence with the proper verb and antecedent agreement:
    Neither of _____ _____ able to finish our supper.
    A. we; were
    B. we; was
    C. us; were
    D. us; was

12. Which word in the following sentence is a noun?
    The library books are overdue.
    A. The
    B. library
    C. books
    D. overdue

13. Which of the following is a simple sentence?
    A. Mary and Samantha ran and skipped and hopped their way home from school every day.
    B. Mary liked to hop but Samantha preferred to skip.
    C. Mary loved coloring yet disliked when coloring was assigned for math homework.
    D. Samantha thought Mary was her best friend but she was mistaken.

14. Which of the following is NOT a simple sentence?
    A. Matthew and Thomas had been best friends since grade school.
    B. Matthew was tall and shy, and Thomas was short and talkative.
    C. Matthew liked to get Thomas to pass notes to the little red-haired girl in the back row of math class.
    D. Matthew and Thomas would tease Mary and Samantha on their way home from school every day.

15. Which of the following sentences is punctuated correctly?
    A. "Theres a bus coming so hurry up and cross the street!" yelled Bob to the old woman.
    B. "There's a bus coming, so hurry up and cross the street", yelled Bob, to the old woman.
    C. "Theres a bus coming, so hurry up and cross the street,"! yelled Bob to the old woman.
    D. "There's a bus coming, so hurry up and cross the street!" yelled Bob to the old_woman.

16. Which of the following sentences is punctuated correctly?
    A. It's a long to-do list she left for us today: make beds, wash breakfast dishes, go grocery shopping, do laundry, cook dinner, and read the twins a bedtime story.

B. Its a long to-do list she left for us today; make beds; wash breakfast dishes; go grocery shopping; do laundry; cook dinner; and read the twins a bedtime story.

C. It's a long to-do list she left for us today: make beds; wash breakfast dishes; go grocery shopping; do laundry; cook dinner; and read the twins a bedtime story.

D. Its a long to-do list she left for us today: make beds, wash breakfast dishes, go grocery shopping, do laundry, cook dinner, and read the twins a bedtime story.

17. Which of the following sentences is written in the first person?
    A. My room was a mess so my mom made me clean it before I was allowed to leave the house.
    B. Her room was a mess so she had to clean it before she left for the concert.
    C. You had better clean up your room before your mom comes home!
    D. Sandy is a slob and never cleans up her own room until her mom makes her.

18. Which sentence follows the rules for capitalization?
    A. My second grade Teacher's name was Mrs. Carmicheal.
    B. The Pope gave a very emotional address to the crowd after Easter Sunday mass.
    C. The president of France is meeting with President Obama later this week.
    D. My family spent our summer vacations at grandpa Joe's cabin in the Finger Lakes region.

19. The girl returning home after her curfew found the _____ up the stairs to her bedroom maddening as it seemed every step she took on the old staircase yielded a loud _____.

    Which of the following completes the sentence above?
    A. clime; creak
    B. clime; creek
    C. climb; creek
    D. climb; creak

20. By this time next summer, _____ my college coursework.
    Which of the following correctly completes the sentence above?
    A. I did complete
    B. I completed
    C. I will complete
    D. I will have completed

21. Which of the following choices best completes this sentence?
    The teacher nodded her _____ to the classroom _____ who was teaching a portion of the daily lesson for the first time.
    A. assent; aide
    B. assent; aid
    C. ascent; aide
    D. ascent; aid

22. Which of the following sentences is grammatically correct?
    A. No one has offered to let us use there home for the office's end-of-year picnic.
    B. No one have offered to let we use their home for the office's end-of-year picnic.
    C. No one has offered to let ourselves use their home for the office's end-of-year picnic.

D. No one has offered to let us use their home for the office's end-of-year picnic.

23. Which choice most effectively combines the information in the following sentences?

The tornado struck. It struck without warning. It caused damage.

The damage was extensive.
   A. Without warning, the extensively damaging tornado struck.
   B. Having struck without warning, the damage was extensive with the tornado.
   C. The tornado struck without warning and caused extensive damage.
   D. Extensively damaging, and without warning, struck the tornado.

24. Which word in the sentence below is a verb?

Carrying heavy boxes to the attic caused her to throw out her back.
   A. Carrying
   B. to
   C. caused
   D. out

25. Which choice below most effectively combines the information in the following sentences?

His lecture was boring. I thought it would never end. My eyelids were drooping. My feet were going numb.
   A. His never-ending lecture made my eyelids droop, and my feet were going numb.
   B. My eyelids drooping and my feet going numb, I thought his boring lecture would never end.
   C. His lecture was boring and would not end; it made my eyelids droop and my feet go numb.
   D. Never-ending, his boring lecture caused me to have droopy eyelids and for my feet to go numb.

26. Which choice below correctly completes this sentence?

Comets _____ balls of dust and ice, _____ leftover materials that _____ planets during the formation of _____ solar system.
   A. Comets is balls of dust and ice, comprised of leftover materials that were not becoming planets during the formation of its solar system.
   B. Comets are balls of dust and ice, comprising leftover materials that are not becoming planets during the formation of our solar system.
   C. Comets are balls of dust and ice, comprised of leftover materials that became planets during the formation of their solar system.
   D. Comets are balls of dust and ice, comprised of leftover materials that did not become planets during the formation of our solar system.

Questions 27-35 are based on the following passage about Penny Dreadfuls.

Victorian era Britain experienced social changes that resulted in increased literacy rates. With the rise of capitalism and industrialization, people began to spend more money on entertainment, contributing to the popularization of the novel. Improvements in printing resulted in the production of newspapers, as well as, Englands' more fully recognizing the singular concept of reading as a form of leisure; it was, of itself, a new industry. An increased capacity for travel via the invention of tracks, engines, and the coresponding railway distribution created both a market for cheap popular literature, and the ability for it to be circulated on a large scale.

The first penny serials were published in the 1830s to meet this demand. The serials were priced to be affordable to working-class readers, and were considerably cheaper than the serialized novels of authors such as Charles Dickens, which cost a shilling (twelve pennies) per part. Those who could not afford a penny a week, working class boys often formed clubs sharing the cost, passed the booklets, who were flimsy, from reader to reader. Other enterprising youngsters would collect a number of consecutive parts, then rent the volume out to friends.

The stories themselves were reprints, or sometimes rewrites, of gothic thrillers, as well as new stories about famous criminals. Other serials were thinly-disguised plagiarisms of popular contemporary literature. The penny dreadfuls were influential since they were in the words of one commentator the most alluring and low-priced form of escapist reading available to ordinary youth.

In reality, the serial novels were overdramatic and sensational, but generally harmless. If anything, the penny dreadfuls, although obviously not the most enlightening or inspiring of literary selections, resulted in increasingly literate youth in the Industrial period. The wide circulation of this sensationalist literature, however, contributed to an ever greater fear of crime in mid-Victorian Britain.

27. Which of the following is the correct punctuation for the following sentence from paragraph 1?
    A. NO CHANGE
    B. Improvements in printing resulted in the production of newspapers, as well as England's more fully recognizing the singular concept of reading as a form of leisure; it was, of itself, a new industry.
    C. Improvements in printing resulted in the production of newspapers, as well as Englands more fully recognizing the singular concept of reading as a form of leisure; it was, of itself, a new industry.
    D. Improvements in printing resulted in the production of newspapers as well as, England's more fully recognizing the singular concept of reading as a form of leisure; it was, of itself, a new industry.

28. In the first sentence of paragraph 1, which of the following words should be capitalized?
    A. era
    B. social
    C. literacy
    D. rates

29. In the last sentence of paragraph 1, which of the following words is misspelled?
    A. capacity
    B. via
    C. coresponding
    D. cheap

30. In the first sentence of the paragraph 2, "this demand" refers to which of the following antecedents in paragraph 1?
    A. travel

B. leisure
C. industry
D. market

31. Which of the following sentences is the clearest way to express the ideas in the third sentence of paragraph 2?
    A. A penny a week, working class boys could not afford these books; they often formed sharing clubs that were passing the flimsy booklets around from one reader to another reader.
    B. Clubs were formed to buy the flimsy booklets by working class boys who could not afford a penny a week that would share the cost, passing from reader to reader the flimsy booklets.
    C. Working class boys who could not afford a penny a week often formed clubs that would share the cost, passing the flimsy booklets from reader to reader.
    D. Sharing the cost were working class boys who could not afford a penny a week; they often formed clubs and, reader to reader, passed the flimsy booklets around.

32. Which word in the first sentence of paragraph 3 should be capitalized?
    A. stories
    B. gothic
    C. thrillers
    D. criminals

33. Which of the following versions of the final sentence of paragraph 3 is correctly punctuated?
    A. The penny dreadfuls were influential since they were in the words of one commentator; the most alluring and low-priced form of escapist reading available to ordinary youth.
    B. The penny dreadfuls were influential since they were, in the words of one commentator, "the most alluring and low-priced form of escapist reading available to ordinary youth".
    C. The penny dreadfuls were influential since they were, in the words of one commentator, the most alluring and low-priced form of escapist reading available to ordinary youth.
    D. The penny dreadfuls were influential since they were in the words of one commentator "the most alluring and low-priced form of escapist reading available to ordinary youth."

34. In this first sentence of paragraph, which of the following words is a noun?
    A. serial
    B. novels
    C. sensational
    D. generally

35. In the last sentence of paragraph, which of the following words is an adjective?
    A. circulation
    B. literature
    C. however
    D. greater

36. The author wants to add a sentence to the passage that would list some of the books which were plagiarized into penny dreadfuls. Which paragraph would be the best place to add this information?
    - A. Paragraph 1
    - B. Paragraph 2
    - C. Paragraph 3
    - D. Paragraph 4

Questions 37-43 are based on the following passage about Martin Luther King Jr.

Martin Luther King Jr. was an American baptist minister and activist who was a leader in the African-American Civil Rights Movement. He is best known for his role in the advancement of civil rights using non-violent civil disobedience based on his Christian beliefs. In the United States, his racial equality efforts, and his staunchly advocating civil rights is among, undoubtedly, culturally the most important contributions made by King to last century's society.

King became a civil rights activist early in his career. In 1955, he led the Montgomery bus boycott, and in 1957 he helped found the Southern Christian Leadership Conference (SCLC), serving as its first president. With the SCLC, King led an unsuccessful 1962 struggle against segregation in Albany, Georgia, and helped organize the 1963 nonviolent protests in Birmingham, Alabama. King also helped to organize the 1963 March on Washington where he delivered his famous I Have a Dream speech. There, he established his reputation as the greatest orator in American history.

On October 14, 1964, King justly received the Nobel Piece Prize for combating racial inequality through nonviolent resistance. In 1965, he helped to organize the famous Selma to Montgomery marches, and the following year he and SCLC took the movement north to Chicago to work on eliminating the unjust and much-despised segregated housing there. In the final years of his life, King expanded his focus to include opposition towards poverty and the Vietnam War, and he gave a famous speech in 1967 entitled "Beyond Vietnam". This speech alienated many of his liberal allies in government who supported the war, but to his credit King never allowed politics to dictate the path of his noble works.

In 1968, King was planning a national occupation of Washington, D.C., to be called the Poor People's Campaign, when he was assassinated on April 4 in Memphis, Tennessee. His violent death was, not surprisingly, followed by riots in many U.S. cities.

King was posthumously awarded the Presidential Medal of Freedom and the Congressional Gold Metal. Martin Luther King, Jr. Day was established as a holiday in numerous cities and states beginning in 1971, and eventually became a U.S. federal holiday in 1986. Since his tragic death, numerous streets in the U.S. have been renamed in his honor, and a county in Washington State was also renamed for him. The Martin Luther King, Jr. Memorial on the National Mall in Washington, D.C., was dedicated in 2011.

37. In the first sentence of paragraph 1, which of the following words should be capitalized?
    - A. baptist
    - B. minister
    - C. activist

    D. leader

38. Which is the best rewording for clarity and concision of this sentence from paragraph 1?
    A. His efforts to achieve racial equality in the United States, and his staunch public advocacy of civil rights are undoubtedly among the most important cultural contributions made to society in the last century.
    B. His efforts achieving equality in the United States, and to staunchly advocate civil rights are undoubtedly among the most important contributions culturally and societally made in the last century.
    C. Racial equality and civil rights, staunchly advocated by King in the United States, are, without a doubt, last century's greatest contributions, in a cultural way, to society.
    D. Last century, King made cultural contributions to racial equality and civil rights, which are undoubtedly the greatest made in the previous century.

39. Which of the following found in paragraph 2 should be placed inside quotation marks?
    A. Montgomery bus boycott
    B. Southern Christian Leadership Conference
    C. March on Washington
    D. I Have a Dream

40. In the first sentence of paragraph 3, which of the following words is misspelled?
    A. received
    B. Piece
    C. combating
    D. racial

41. In the first sentence of paragraph 5, which of the following words is misspelled?
    A. Posthumously
    B. Presidential
    C. Medal
    D. Metal

42. Which of the following sentences from the passage provides context clues about the author's feelings in regard to King?
    A. He is best known for his role in the advancement of civil rights using non-violent civil disobedience based on his Christian beliefs. (P. 1)
    B. King also helped to organize the 1963 March on Washington where he delivered his famous I Have a Dream speech. (P. 2)
    C. This speech alienated many of his liberal allies in government who supported the war, but to his credit King never allowed politics to dictate the path of his noble works. (P. 3)
    D. King was posthumously awarded the Presidential Medal of Freedom and the Congressional Gold Metal. (P. 5)

43. The author is considering adding a paragraph about King's family to the passage. Should he or she do this?
    A. Yes, because it adds needed personal details to the passage.

B. Yes, because it would elaborate on information already provided in the passage.

C. No, because the passage is about King's public life and works, and information about his family would be irrelevant.

D. No, because information about his family has already been included and an additional paragraph on that topic would be redundant.

44. Which of the following sentences uses correct punctuation for dialogue?

A. "Hey, can you come here a second"? asked Marie.

B. She thought about his offer briefly and then responded. "I think I will have to pass".

C. "I am making pancakes for breakfast. Does anybody want some?" asked mom.

D. The conductor yelled "All aboard"! and then waited for last minute travelers to board the train.

45. Which of the following is a compound sentence?

A. She and I drove to the play together.

B. I woke up early that morning and began to do long-neglected household chores.

C. The long-separated cousins ran and jumped and sang and played all afternoon.

D. I trembled when I saw him: his face was white as a ghost.

46. Which of the following is the best order for the sentences below in forming a logical paragraph?

A. A, B, C, D, E

B. A, C, E, B, D

C. A, D, B, D, E

D. A, C, E, D, B

A. *Walt Disney was a shy, self-deprecating and insecure man in private but adopted a warm and outgoing public persona.*

B. *His film work continues to be shown and adapted; his studio maintains high standards in its production of popular entertainment, and the Disney amusement parks have grown in size and number to attract visitors in several countries.*

C. *However he had high standards and high expectations of those with whom he worked.*

D. *He nevertheless remains an important figure in the history of animation and in the cultural history of the United States, where he is considered a national cultural icon.*

E. *His reputation changed in the years after his death, from a purveyor of homely patriotic values to a representative of American imperialism.*

47. Which of the choices below is the meaning of the word "adopted" in the following sentence?

Walt Disney was a shy, self-deprecating and insecure man in private but adopted a warm and outgoing public persona.

A. took

B. began to use

C. began to have

D. legally cared for as one's own child

48. Which of the following sentences is written in the second person?

A. You had better call and RSVP to the party right away before you forget.

B. She had every intention of calling with a prompt reply to the invitation, but the week got hectic and she forgot.

C. I am utterly hopeless at remembering things, so I will set up a calendar reminder for myself to call Jan about the party.

D. "Did you forget to RSVP to the party?!" asked her exasperated roommate.

49. Which of the following sentences shows proper pronoun-antecedent agreement?
    A. The author published several best-selling novels; some of it was made into films that were not as popular.
    B. Everyone should bring their parents to the town-wide carnival.
    C. Smart companies will do what it takes to hold onto its best employees.
    D. Parents are reminded to pick up their children from school promptly at 2:30.

50. Which of the following sentences shows proper subject-verb agreement?
    A. Danny is one of the only students who have lived up to his responsibilities as a newspaper staff member.
    B. One of my friends are going to be on a TV series starting this fall.
    C. Rice and beans, my favorite meal, reminds me of my native country Puerto Rico.
    D. Most of the milk we bought for the senior citizens' luncheons have gone bad.

51. Which sentence below illustrates proper use of punctuation for dialogue?
    A. "I have a dream", began Martin Luther King, Jr.
    B. "Can you believe that I have been asked to audition for that part," asked Megan excitedly?
    C. "You barely know him! How can she marry him?" was the worried mother's response at her teenager's announcement of marriage.
    D. "Remain seated while the seatbelt signs are illuminated." Came the announcement over the airplane's loud speaker system.

52. Which of the sentences below is NOT in the second person?
    A. "I have a dream", began Martin Luther King, Jr.
    B. "Can you believe that I have been asked to audition for that part," asked Megan excitedly?
    C. "You barely know him! How can you marry him?" was the worried mother's response at her teenager's announcement of marriage.
    D. "Remain seated while the seatbelt signs are illuminated." Came the announcement over the airplane's loud speaker system.

53. Which of the following sentences is an example of an Imperative sentence?
    A. "I have a dream", began Martin Luther King, Jr.

B. "Can you believe that I have been asked to audition for that part," asked Megan excitedly?

C. "You barely know him! How can she marry him?" was the worried mother's response at her teenager's announcement of marriage.

D. "Please remain seated while the seatbelt signs are illuminated." Came the announcement over the airplane's loud speaker system.

54. Which of the following means "the act of cutting out"?
   A. Incision
   B. Concision
   C. Excision
   D. Decision

55. Which of the following refers to an inflammation?
   A. Appendectomy
   B. Colitis
   C. Angioplasty
   D. Dermatology

56. Which of the following refers to a cancer?
   A. Neuropathy
   B. Hysterectomy
   C. Oncology
   D. Melanoma

57. Which of the following conditions is associated with the nose?
   A. Hematoma
   B. Neuralgia
   C. Rhinitis
   D. Meningitis

58. Which of the following refers to the study of something?
   A. Gastroenterology
   B. Gastritis
   C. Psychosis
   D. Psychopath

ADVANCED PRACTICE TEST: ENGLISH

Passage 1

The United States Treasury operates a subsidiary, the Bureau of Engraving and Printing (BEP), where the nation's supply of paper money is designed and manufactured. But to call American currency "paper" money is a slight misnomer that understates its unperceived complexity and intrinsic technological sophistication. The Treasury goes to extraordinary lengths to safeguard cash from counterfeiters. One of the most fundamental ways is by printing not on paper, per se, but on a proprietary blend of linen and cotton. American money is more akin to fabric than paper, and each bill that is printed is a phenomenal work of art and masterful craftsmanship.

The most frequently counterfeited denominations are the 20-dollar bill, preferred by domestic counterfeiters, and the 100-dollar note, which is the currency of choice for foreign forgers. To make the copying of twenties more difficult, the BEP uses color-shifting ink that changes from copper to green in certain lights. Evidence of this can be seen in the numeral "20" located in the lower right corner on the front of the bills. A portrait watermark – which is a very faint, rather ethereal image of President Jackson – is also juxtaposed into the blank space to the right to his visible and prominent portrait. Additionally, there is a security ribbon, adorned with a flag and the words "USA Twenty," printed on and embedded into the bill. When exposed to ultraviolet light, the thread glows with a greenish hue. Twenties also include an almost subliminal text that reads "USA20;" this micro-printed text is well-camouflaged within the bill. With the use of a magnifying glass, it can be found in the border beneath the Treasurer's signature.

The 100-dollar bill utilizes similar security features. These include color-shifting ink, portrait watermarks, security threads and ribbons, raised printing, and micro-printing. These units of currency, dubbed "Ben Franklins" in honor of the president whose face graces it, also boast what the BEP describes as a 3-D security ribbon. The ribbon has bells and numbers printed on it. When the currency is tilted it appears that the images of bells transform into the numeral 100 and, when tilted side to side, the bells and 100s seem to move in a lateral direction.

Security threads woven into each different denomination have their own respective colors, and each one glows a different color when illuminated with ultraviolet light. Fine engraving or printing patterns appear in various locations on bills too, and many of these patterns are extremely fine. The artists who create them for engraving also incorporate non-linear designs, as the waviness can make it exponentially more difficult to successfully counterfeit the currency. The surface of American currency is also slightly raised, giving it a subtly, but distinct, tactile characteristic.

1. Which of the following conclusions may logically be drawn from the first paragraph of the passage?
   A. Linen and cotton are more expensive printing materials than paper.
   B. The current process of printing money is reflective of decades of modifications.
   C. Counterfeiting of American money is an enormous problem.
   D. The artistry inherent in the making of American money makes it attractive to collectors.

2. What sentence, if added to the end of the passage, would provide the best conclusion to both the paragraph and the passage?
   A. It is clear from all these subtly nuanced features of the various bills that true artistry is at work in their making.
   B. Yet, despite all of these technological innovations, the race to stay ahead of savvy counterfeiters and their constantly changing counterfeiting techniques is a never-ending one.
   C. Due to the complexities involved in the printing of money, these artists are consequently well-paid for their skills.

  D. Thus, many other countries have begun to model their money-printing methods on these effective techniques.

3. The passage is reflective of which of the following types of writing?
  A. Descriptive
  B. Narrative
  C. Expository
  D. Persuasive

4. This passage likely comes from which of the following documents?
  A. A pamphlet for tourists visiting the United States Treasury
  B. A feature news article commemorating the bicentennial of the Bureau of Engraving and Printing
  C. A letter from the US treasury Secretary to the President
  D. A public service message warning citizens about the increased circulation of counterfeit currency

5. Which of the following is an example of a primary source document?
  A. A pamphlet for tourists visiting the United States Treasury
  B. A feature news article commemorating the bicentennial of the Bureau of Engraving and Printing
  C. A letter from the US treasury Secretary to the President
  D. A public service message warning citizens about the increased circulation of counterfeit currency

6. Which of the following describes the word *intrinsic* as it is used in the first paragraph of the passage?
  A. Amazing
  B. Expensive
  C. Unbelievable
  D. Inherent

Passage 2

In the Middle Ages, merchants an artisans formed groups called "guilds" to protect themselves and their trades. Guilds appeared in the year 1000, and by the twelfth century, analogous trades, like wool, spice, and silk dealers had formed their own guilds. _____, towns like Florence, Italy, boasted as many as 50 merchants' guilds. With the advent of guilds, apprenticeship became a complex system. Apprentices were to be taught only certain things and then they were to prove they possessed certain skills, as determined by the guild. Each guild decided the length of time required for an apprentice to work for a master tradesman before being admitted to the trade.

7. The topic sentence of the above passage is
  A. In the Middle Ages, merchants an artisans formed groups called "guilds" to protect themselves and their trades.
  B. Guilds appeared in the year 1000, and by the twelfth century, analogous trades, like wool, spice, and silk dealers had formed their own guilds.
  C. With the advent of guilds, apprenticeship became a complex system.

D. Apprentices were to be taught only certain things and then they were to prove they possessed certain skills, as determined by the guild.

8. The main idea of the passage is that
   A. wool, spice and silk dealers were all types of merchant trades during the Middle Ages.
   B. Florence, Italy was a great center of commerce during the Middle Ages.
   C. merchant guilds originated in the Middle Ages and became extremely popular, eventually leading to a sophisticated apprenticeship system.
   D. apprenticeships were highly sought after, therefore merchants had many skilled workers to choose from to assist them in their trade.

9. From the content of the passage, it reasonably be inferred that
   A. prior to the inception of guilds, merchants were susceptible to competition from lesser skilled craftsmen peddling inferior products or services.
   B. most merchants were unscrupulous business who often cheated their customers.
   C. it was quite easy to become an apprentice to a highly skilled merchant.
   D. guilds fell out of practice during the Industrial Revolution due to the mechanization of labor.

10. As it is used in the second sentence, "analogous" most nearly means
    A. obsolete
    B. inferior
    C. similar
    D. less popular

11. Which of the following is the best signal word or phrase to fill in the blank above?
    A. Up until that time,
    B. Before that time,
    C. By that time,
    D. After that time,

Passage 3

Certainly we must face this fact: if the American press, as a mass medium, has formed the minds of America, the mass has also formed the medium. There is action, reaction, and interaction going on ceaselessly between the newspaper-buying public and the editors. What is wrong with the American press is what is in part wrong with American society. Is this, _____, to exonerate the American press for its failures to give the American people more tasteful and more illuminating reading matter? Can the American press seek to be excused from responsibility for public lack of information as TV and radio often do, on the grounds that, after all, "we have to give the people what they want or we will go out of business"?   --Clare Boothe Luce

12. What is the primary purpose of this text?
    A. To reveal an innate problem in American society
    B. To criticize the American press for not taking responsibility for their actions
    C. To analyze the complex relationship that exists between the public and the media
    D. To challenge the masses to protest the lack of information disseminated by the media

13. From which of the following is the above paragraph most likely excerpted?
    A. A newspaper editorial letter
    B. A novel about yellow journalism
    C. A diary entry
    D. A speech given at a civil rights protest

14. Which of the following is an example of a primary source document?
    A. A newspaper editorial letter
    B. A novel about yellow journalism
    C. A diary entry
    D. A speech given at a civil rights protest

15. As it is used in sentence 4, "illuminating" most nearly means
    A. intelligent
    B. sophisticated
    C. interesting
    D. enlightening

16. Which of the following is the best signal word or phrase to fill in the blank?
    A. so
    B. however
    C. therefore
    D. yet

17. What is the author's primary attitude towards the American press?
    A. admiration
    B. perplexity
    C. disapproval
    D. ambivalence

18. Which of the following identifies the mode of the passage?
    A. expository
    B. persuasive/argumentative
    C. narrative
    D. descriptive

19. Based on the passage, which of the following can most likely be concluded?
    A. The author has a degree in journalism
    B. The author has worked in the journalism industry
    C. The author is seeking employment at a newspaper
    D. The author is filing a lawsuit against a media outlet

Passage 4

The game today known as "football" in the United States can be traced directly back to the English game of rugby, although there have been many changes to the game. Football was played informally on university fields more than a hundred years ago. In 1840, a yearly series of informal "scrimmages" started at Yale University. It took more than twenty-five years, _____, for the game to become a part of college life. The first formal intercollegiate football game was held between Princeton and Rutgers teams on November 6, 1869 on Rutgers' home field at New Brunswick, New Jersey, and Rutgers won.

20. Which sentence, if added to the end of the paragraph, would provide the best conclusion?
    A. Despite an invitation to join the Ivy League, Rutgers University declined, but later joined the Big Ten Conference instead.
    B. Football was played for decades on school campuses nationwide before the American Professional Football Association was formed in 1920, and then renamed the National Football League (or the NFL) two years later.
    C. Women were never allowed to play football, and that fact remains a controversial policy at many colleges and universities.
    D. Football remains the national pastime, despite rising popularity for the game of soccer, due to increased TV coverage of World Cup matches.

21. Which of the following is the best signal word or phrase to fill in the blank above?
    A. however
    B. still
    C. in addition
    D. alternatively

Passage 5

Modernism is a philosophical movement that arose during the early 20th century. Among the factors that shaped modernism were the development of modern societies based on industry and the rapid growth of cities, followed later by the horror of World War I. Modernism rejected the science-based thinking of the earlier Era of Enlightenment, and many modernists also rejected religion. The poet Ezra Pound's 1934 injunction to "Make it new!" was the touchstone of the movement's approach towards what it saw as the now obsolete culture of the past. A notable characteristic of modernism is self-consciousness and irony concerning established literary and social traditions, which often led to experiments concerned with HOW things were made, not so much with the actual final product. Modernism had a profound impact on numerous aspects of life, and its values and perspectives still influence society in many positive ways today.

22. According to the passage, what is the overarching theme of the modernist movement?
    A. Rejection of the past and outmoded ideas
    B. Appreciation of urban settings over natural settings
    C. A concentration on method over form
    D. A focus on automated industry

23. As it is used in the passage, "touchstone" most nearly means
    A. Challenge
    B. Basis
    C. Fashion
    D. Metaphor

24. Which of the following statements from the passage can be described as an opinion?

A. Among the factors that shaped modernism were the development of modern societies based on industry and the rapid growth of cities, followed later by the horror of World War I.

B. The poet Ezra Pound's 1934 injunction to "Make it new!" was the touchstone of the movement's approach towards what it saw as the now obsolete culture of the past.

C. A notable characteristic of modernism is self-consciousness and irony concerning established literary and social traditions, which often led to experiments concerned with HOW things were made, not so much with the actual final product.

D. Modernism had a profound impact on numerous aspects of life, and its values and perspectives still influence society in many positive ways today.

Passage 6

The modern Olympics are the leading international sporting event featuring summer and winter sports competitions in which thousands of athletes from around the world participate in a variety of competitions. Held every two years, with the Summer and Winter Games alternating, the games are a modern way to bring nations together, _____ allowing for national pride, and sportsmanship on a global scale. Having withstood the test of time over many centuries, they are the best example of the physical achievements of mankind.

The creation of the modern Games was inspired by the ancient Olympic Games, which were held in Olympia, Greece, from the 8th century BC to the 4th century AD. The Ancient Games events were fewer in number and were examples of very basic traditional forms of competitive athleticism. Many running events were featured, as well as a pentathlon (consisting of a jumping event, discus and javelin throws, a foot race, and wrestling), boxing, wrestling, *pankration*, and equestrian events. Fast forward to the modern state of this ancient athletic competition, and we see that the Olympic Movement during the 20th and 21st centuries has resulted in several changes to the Games, including the creation of the Winter Olympic Games for ice and winter sports, which for climate reasons, would not have been possible in ancient Greece. The Olympics has also shifted away from pure amateurism to allowing participation of professional athletes, a change which was met with criticism when first introduced, as many felt it detracted from the original spirit and intention of the competition.

Today, over 13,000 athletes compete at the summer and Winter Olympic Games in 33 different sports and nearly 400 events. The first, second, and third-place finishers in each event receive Olympic medals: gold, silver, and bronze, respectively. And every country hopes to be able to go home with many of these medals, as they are truly still a point of pride for each nation to be recognized for some outstanding achievement on the world stage, however briefly.

25. Which of the following is the best signal word or phrase to fill in the blank in the first paragraph?
    A. despite
    B. however
    C. instead of
    D. as well as

26. Which of the following words from the last sentence of paragraph 2 has a negative connotation?
    A. Shifted

B. Allowing

C. Change

D. Detracted

27. Which of the following statements based on the passage would be considered an opinion?
    A. The ancient Olympic games were held in Olympia, Greece.
    B. The Olympic games are the best example of humanity's physical prowess.
    C. When the games were changed from pure amateurism to allowing professional athletes to participate, this change displeased many people.
    D. Today, 33 different sports are represented at the Olympic games.

Passage 7

A day or two later, in the afternoon, I saw myself staring at my fire, at an inn which I had booked on foreseeing that I would spend some weeks in London. I had just come in, and, having decided on a spot for my luggage, sat down to consider my room. It was on the ground floor, and the fading daylight reached it in a sadly broken-down condition. It struck me that the room was stuffy and unsocial, with its moldy smell and its decoration of lithographs and waxy flowers – it seemed an impersonal black hole in the huge general blackness of the inn itself. The uproar of the neighborhood outside hummed away, and the rattle of a heartless hansom cab passed close to my ears. A sudden horror of the whole place came over me, like a tiger-pounce of homesickness which had been watching its moment. London seemed hideous, vicious, cruel and, above all, overwhelming. Soon, I would have to go out for my dinner, and it appeared to me that I would rather remain dinnerless, would rather even starve, than go forth into the hellish town where a stranger might get trampled to death, and have his carcass thrown into the Thames River.

28. Based on the passage above, the author's attitude toward his experience in London can best be described as
    A. Awe
    B. Disappointment
    C. Revulsion
    D. Ambivalence

29. Which type of document is this passage likely excerpted from?
    A. A travel guide
    B. A diary entry
    C. A news editorial
    D. An advertisement

30. Which of the following documents would likely NOT be considered a primary source document?
    A. A travel guide
    B. A diary entry
    C. A news editorial
    D. An advertisement

31. Based on the content of the passage, which of the following is a reasonable conclusion?
    A. The author is quite wealthy.
    B. The author has been to London before.

C. The author is traveling to London based on the recommendation of a friend.
D. The author will not be traveling to London again.

BASIC PRACTICE TEST: SCIENCE

1- C. Convection currents in the Earth's mantle layer

The temperature of the Earth's interior increases as one approaches the Earth's core and decreases as one nears the surface. Since heat rises, this temperature difference between deeper and shallower regions of the Earth generates convection currents in the Earth's mantle that carries heat from the interior of the Earth toward the surface. Near the surface of the Earth, the rising plumes of mantle reach the Earth's crust, and spread outward beneath the Earth's tectonic plates. The plates are carried along the Earth's surface by the surface motion of these mantle convection currents.

2- B. The moon completes one full central-axis rotation in the same amount of time that it completes one full orbit of the Earth

This is a concept that is easier to observe with three-dimensional models of the moon in orbit around the Earth. If an object completes one full rotation around its central axis in the same amount of time that it completes one full rotation around another object, the result is that the orbiting object must always present the same face to the object that it is orbiting. This type of orbit is common in the solar system and the term for this relationship is tidal locking. The moon is tidally locked in its orbit around the Earth.

3- B. Is directly proportional to the object's mass

The force of gravity between two objects, m_1 and m_2, is proportional to the product of the two masses divided by the distance squared between the centers of mass of the two objects, d^2. On the surface of the Earth, m_1 is the object mass and m_2 is the Earth's mass, m_e. The formula is $F_g=G(m_1{}_*m_e/d^2)$. G is the gravitational constant. It is clear from this formula that as an object's mass increases, the force of gravity increases. If the mass doubles, the force of gravity doubles. This is a directly proportional relationship between mass and the force of gravity. For an object on the surface of the Earth, the distance between the object's center of mass and the Earth's center of mass is very close to the radius of the Earth. If this distance doubles by locating the mass one additional Earth radius away from the Earth's center, the formula for the force of gravity shows that the gravitational force on the mass will decrease by a factor of 4, since the force of gravity is inversely proportional to the square of the distance between the centers of the two objects. The force of gravity on the object one Earth radius above the surface of the Earth will be ¼ of the force of gravity that the object experiences at the surface of the Earth.

4- A. The direction that electrons flow through a circuit reverses at a fixed rate of electron flow direction per unit time for alternating current. The direction that electrons flow through a circuit remains constant for direct current.

Alternating current is electron flow that reverses at a regular rate when traveling through an electrically conductive pathway, such as an electrical wire in a circuit, or in electrical power lines. Direct current is electron flow that does not change its direction of flow over time when traveling through an electrically conductive pathway. Alternating current is a much safer and more efficient means of generating and distributing electricity. In the United States, the electrical power grid uses alternating current that switches direction 60 times per second.

5- D.   Class and Division

The biological classification hierarchy for organisms is Genus, Family, Order, Class, Phylum/Division, Kingdom, Domain. Therefore, all species that are members of the same order must also be members of the higher levels of the classification system, namely the same Class, Phylum/Division, Kingdom and Domain.

6- D.   The same atomic number

All of the atoms of a given element have the same number of protons. This number of protons is equal to the atomic number for a given element. There are a unique number of protons that correspond to every atomic element. Atoms of the same element can have different numbers of neutrons. Neutrons and protons are both nucleons, so different atoms of the same element may also have different numbers of nucleons. The atomic mass of an atom is nearly equal to the sum of the masses of the atom's nucleus, so different atoms of an element may have different individual atomic masses.

7- A.   1 newton (N) times 1 meter (m)

The joule is an SI unit of energy. The SI units of energy can be derived from Newton's laws of motion. The energy of motion transferred to an object is equal to the force (F) applied to an object in the object's direction of motion times the distance (d) over which the force is applied. This can be stated as the general equation that energy equals force times distance, $E=(F)(d)$. The SI unit of force is the newton (N), which has units of $kg\text{-}m^2s^{-2}$. Since the SI unit for distance is the meter, the SI unit for energy, the joule, can be written as the SI unit for force, the newton, times 1 meter. This may also be expressed as one newton-meter or 1 N-m.

8- B.   A bilayer of phospholipid molecules

All biological cells, both prokaryotic and eukaryotic, have a phospholipid molecule bilayer cell membrane structure. The individual molecules are long-chain hydrocarbons with a phosphate group chemically bonded at one end of each molecule. In an aqueous (water-rich) environment, these molecules will naturally form bilayer bubble structures with the electrically charged phosphate groups facing outward on the outer layer and inward on the inner layer. The uncharged lipid tails of the molecules face toward the center of the bilayer.

9- D.   3.0 to 2.0

The pH of a solution is equal to the negative log of the hydrogen ion concentration of the solution. HCl is a strong acid that completely dissociates in an aqueous solution, forming one hydrogen ion (H^+) and one chloride ion (Cl^-) per HCl molecule. A 5×10^{-3} M solution of hydrochloric acid will therefore produce a solution that has a 5×10^{-3} M hydrogen ion concentration. 5×10^{-3} M is between 1×10^{-3} M, which is equivalent to a pH of 3, and 1×10^{-2} M, which is equivalent to a pH of 2.

10- D.   400 N

The equation for the force required to maintain an object in unchanging circular motion is $F_c=(mv^2)/r$, where, in this case, m=the mass of the ball, r=the length of the rope and v= the tangential velocity of the ball. Therefore $F_c=(0.5\ kg)(20\ m\text{-}s^{-1})^2/(0.5\ m)$; this simplifies to 400 $kg\text{-}m\text{-}s^{-2}$. Notice that $kg\text{-}m\text{-}s^-$

^{2} are the units for newtons; the SI units of force required to maintain this type of motion is 400 newtons (400 N).

11-C. Pupil dilation and bronchial dilation

The sympathetic nervous system is the "fight or flight" response division of the autonomic nervous system. The parasympathetic nervous system is the "rest and digest" division of the autonomic nervous system. Sympathetic physiological effects include pupil dilation – which enhances visual acuity, bronchial dilation – which increases the efficiency and maximum rate of air exchange of the respiratory system and suppression of digestion – which allows blood flow and energy consumption to be redirected from digestive activities to physiological activities required during fight or flight situations.

12-A. A continued normal evolution of the present ecosystem

There have been five mass extinctions in Earth's history; none have been correlated with a reversal of the Earth's magnetic field. The Earth's magnetic field reverses every few hundred thousand years and there is no evidence of any significant effect to the Earth's ecosystem during such pole reversal events. In fact, there is strong evidence that a pole reversal is happening right now. Scientists estimate the current pole reversal will be complete between 100 and 1000 years from now.

13-D. Fusion of hydrogen atoms

The sun is composed almost entirely of hydrogen and helium. The enormous mass of the sun generates forces of gravity at the core of the sun high enough to cause hydrogen nuclei (protons) to fuse together to form helium nuclei. This fusion reaction generates an incredibly large amount of energy. Fission occurs when a large atomic nucleus such as uranium or plutonium splits apart in two smaller atomic nuclei. This type of reaction does not occur on the sun.

14-A. 15 N/m$_1$

The fundamental equation relating force, mass and acceleration is F=ma, therefore, a=F/m. Substituting the value of 15 N for F gives the acceleration of the object as a =15 N/m$_1$. Notice that this is the general equation for the acceleration due to a specific magnitude of force acting on an object with an unknown mass. The precise value for the acceleration of the mass depends on the magnitude of the mass. For instance, if the mass of the object, m$_1$ is equal to 15 kg, the velocity of the object would be 15 N/15 kg = 1 meter/(second)^2.

15-B. 20 amperes (20 A)

Ohm's law states that, in an electric circuit, the voltage of the circuit is equal to the current of the circuit and the total resistance of the circuit, or V=(I)(R). To solve for the current in the question above, rearrange the equation to solve for the current "I". I=V/R. This gives I=(5 V)/(0.25 Ω); I=20 V/Ω; I=20 amperes or 20 A. Notice that the units for current, amperes (A), is equal to the units for voltage, volts (V) divided by resistance, ohms (Ω).

16-C. The trait's gene likely has two alleles, one that is recessive and one that is dominant.

The question can be explained by using the example of blue and brown eye color in humans. The physical trait is the color of a person's eyes. This trait is determined by a single gene. Every person has two copies of this gene. There are two different alleles or variations of this gene, the brown-eye allele

"B", which is dominant, and the blue-eye allele "b" which is recessive. If a person has at least one brown eye allele out of their pair of eye color genes – "BB" or "Bb", they will have brown eyes as a physical trait. If both parents are "Bb" or heterozygous for eye color, they will each have brown eyes but statistically one in four of their offspring will receive the recessive b allele from each parent. These offspring will have two recessive alleles for eye color, "bb", and will have the physical trait of blue eyes.

17- D.   1,000,000

The volume of a cube is equal to the length times the height times the width of the cube. One meter is 100 centimeters. Therefore the length, width and height of a 1-meter cube is 100 centimeters per side. This gives 100 x 100 x 100 = 1,000,000 cubic centimeters per cubic meter.

18- A.   White dwarf

The fate of stars with stellar masses less than about 1.4 times the mass of our sun is to eventually shrink down to a stellar object known as a white dwarf. Much more massive stars than the sun will eventually explode as supernovae, leaving either a neutron star or a black hole as a remnant of this explosion. A red giant is a stage that the sun will pass through, but not the final stage.

19- C.   A sound wave's maximum velocity is less than a light wave's maximum velocity?

Sound waves require transmission through the movement of matter. Matter can never travel as fast as the maximum speed of a light wave. This is an absolute law of physics.

20- A.   A simple concave mirror

Among simple mirrors and lenses, only mirrors can reflect light rays, as described in the question, back to a point in front of their optical surface. Light rays as described will be reflected inward to a focal point by a concave mirror. A convex mirror will reflect light rays outward in a manner that makes it appear that the rays are originating from a focal point behind the optical surface of the mirror.

21- A.   Slow down and bend toward the perpendicular line

When light crosses from a substance with a lower index of refraction to one with a higher index of refraction, the light slows and bends toward a normal line. A normal line is defined as the perpendicular line described in the question.

22- B.   Mercury, Mars, Venus

The relative size of the planets, beginning with the smallest, is Mercury, Mars, Venus, Earth, Neptune, Uranus, Saturn and Jupiter.

23- D.   Filtration and dilution

Physical changes to molecular compounds will not change the atomic composition or atomic arrangements of molecular compounds. In reductions and oxidations, molecular compounds gain or lose electrons, which is a chemical change. Deprotonation of a compound results in a loss of a proton, also a chemical change. The other events will not result in chemical changes to molecular compounds.

24- C.   4.5

The atomic weight of an element is the average atomic mass of the atoms of the element. In this hypothetical case, helium has two protons; 50% of the atoms have a mass of 4, this being the isotope with the same number of protons and neutrons, and 50% of the atoms have a mass of 5, this being the isotope that has one more neutron than protons. The average of this mixture of atoms is $(4 + 5)/2 = 4.5$.

25- B.   Electromagnetic energy derived from the absorption of photons

The chloroplast is the cellular organelle that allows a cell to carry out photosynthesis. This process is powered by the absorption of photons by chemicals located inside the chloroplast.

26- B.   A gun will experience a force of magnitude 5 N at the same instant that it fires a 5-g bullet that experiences an initial acceleration of 1000 m/s

Newton's 3rd law of motion states that, for every action, there is an equal and opposite reaction. The force required to fire a 5-g bullet with an acceleration of 1000 m/s^2 is F=ma, where m is the mass of the bullet. This gives F= (0.005 kg)(1000 m/s^2) = 5 N. Therefore the gun must experience an equal magnitude and opposite direction force of 5 N at the instant that the bullet is fired.

27- A.   R$_2$ and R$_3$ are connected in parallel

Choice B is incorrect because the total resistance for resistors in series is the sum of the individual resistors, and this would give a total resistance of 10 + 4 + 2 = 16 Ω. Choice c is incorrect because the total resistance, R$_T$, for resistors in parallel is given by the equations $1/R_T = (1/R_1) + (1/R_2) + (1/R_3)$... This gives $1/R_T = (1/10) + (1/4) + (1/2)$; $1/R_T = 17/20$; $R_T = 1\ 3/20$ Ω. The remaining choices describe two resistors in parallel. The remaining resistor can be connected in series with these two resistors. These are complex circuits. First the resistance of the resistors in parallel is calculated with the formula $1/R_T = (1/R_1) + (1/R_2) + (1/R_3)$..., then this resistance is added to the resistance of the remaining resistor since it is connected in series with the two parallel resistors. For choice A, this gives 1/(¼ + ½) = 1 ⅓ Ω for the resistors in parallel. The final resistor R$_1$ = 10 Ω, so the total resistance is 1 ⅓ Ω + 10 Ω = 11 ⅓ Ω.

28- C.   3s orbital

The ranking of electron orbital energy levels, up to the level of the 3d orbitals and beginning with the lowest-energy orbital is 1s, 2s, 2p, 3s, 3d, 3p. In the lowest electron energy state, atoms fill the lower energy orbitals before they begin to add electrons to higher-energy orbitals.

29- B.   The total momentum and kinetic energy of the objects before and after the collision has not changed

When collisions between objects are perfectly elastic, both the total momentum and total kinetic energy of the objects is conserved. This is in contrast to inelastic collisions, where momentum is conserved, but kinetic energy is not conserved.

30- C.   Performed no work on the barbell

To perform work on the barbell, the barbell must be displaced (moved a certain distance) from its initial position by a force acting on the barbell. This is shown by the equation for mechanical work W = Fd. Since the barbell remains motionless during this time, no work is performed on the barbell.

31- A.   140 miles

The equation to determine the distance traveled by an object that is undergoing a constant acceleration is $d = V_o t + \frac{1}{2}(at^2)$, V_o is the object's initial velocity and t is the total time during which the object is accelerating. Plugging in the values stated in the question gives $d = $ (60 miles/hour)(2 hours) + $\frac{1}{2}$(10 miles/hour^2)(2 hours)^2. This gives 120 miles + 20 miles = 140 miles.

32- D.   Remain unchanged

Newton's universal law of gravitation is $F_g = G(m_1)(m_2)/R^2$. For an object with a given mass on the surface of the Earth, its weight is the force of gravity due to the Earth. The formula shows that increasing the Earth's mass by a factor of 4 increases the gravitational force by a factor of 4. Gravitational force is inversely proportional to the square of the Earth's radius. Increasing the radius of the Earth by a factor of 2 will decrease the gravitational force by a factor of 4. Overall, the two effects cancel each other out and there is no net change in the force of gravity and therefore no change in the weight of an object on the surface of the Earth.

33- C.   Increase the object's velocity by 2 m/s and decrease its mass by 950 g

The kinetic energy of an object, "KE", is equal to one-half of the mass of the object multiplied by the square of the object's velocity, $KE = \frac{1}{2}(mv^2)$. The question can be answered by considering that KE is directly proportional to the object's mass and directly proportional to the square of the object's velocity. In choice A, only the mass increases and by a factor less than 2 so the kinetic energy increase is less than twice the original KE. In choice B, the velocity doubles, so this increases the KE by a factor of 4. The mass decreases by an amount less than half and the original mass, so the KE decreases by less than half due to the decreased mass. Overall, the KE increases by a factor greater than 2 but less than 4. In choice D, the velocity increases by a factor less than 2 and the mass doubles (increases by a factor of 2); therefore the KE increases by a factor greater than 2 but less than 4. For choice C, the velocity triples (increases by a factor of 3), which gives a KE increase of three squared, or 9. The mass decreases by a factor of 4. Overall, this gives an increase in KE of a factor of 9-4=5. Therefore in choice C, the object's KE quintuples.

34- C.   800 m/s^2

The formula for acceleration in uniform circular motion or centripetal acceleration is $A_c = V^2/R$. For this question, $A_c = $ (40 m/s)^2 /2 m = 800 m/s^2.

35- A. $M_e = (F_g)(R_{es})^2/(G)(M_s)$

This question requires the knowledge that Newton's law of universal gravitation is $F_g = G(m_1)(m_2)/R^2$. Assign R_{es} as the value for R and the masses of the Earth and sun for m_1 and m_2, Rearrange the equation to solve for the mass of the Earth. This will give the equation $M_e = (F_g)(R_{es})^2/(G)(M_s)$.

36- D.   -13 1/3 m/s

The question describes an inelastic collision between two objects. With no outside forces affecting their velocities, the total momentum of the initial two-object system remains constant before and after the collision. This is the law of conservation of linear momentum. The momentum of an object is equal to an object's mass multiplied by the object's velocity. The momentum of the system before the collision is $(M_A)(V_A) + (M_B)(V_B)$. This gives (1 kg)(20 m/s) + (2 kg)(-30 m/s) = -40 kg-m/s. The final momentum of the system is equal to the sum of masses of A and B multiplied by the resulting velocity of the new two-mass object, "AB": $(M_A + M_B)(V_r)$. Since the momentum of the system remains constant, $(M_A + M_B)(V_r)$ = -40 kg-m/s. Rearrange the equation to solve for V_r, V_r = (-40 kg-m/s)/(1kg +2kg). This gives (-40 kg-m/s)/3 kg = -13 1/3 m/s.

37- C.   One or more mobile valence electrons per atom

An electrical conductor must be able to transfer electrons from one atom to another. Only valence electrons are likely to be transferred by atoms. If every atom has at least one mobile valence electron, by definition these atoms should be able to transfer electrons from one atom to the other.

38- B.   150 N

The equation to determine the force required to overcome the static friction of a surface is F = (Fnormal)(coefficient of static friction). Fnormal is the magnitude of the force that is directed through the object perpendicular to the friction surface. In this case, the force is due to gravity, which is perpendicular to a horizontal surface. This force is given by the equation F = ma, where m is the mass of the object and a is the acceleration due to gravity. This gives Fnormal = (10 kg)(10 m/s^2) = 100 N. In addition to the force required to overcome friction, an additional force in the horizontal direction must also be applied to accelerate the object by a value of 5 m/s squared. Again, use F = ma and solve for an acceleration of 5 m/s^2, F = (10 kg)(5 m/s^2) = 50 N. So 50 + 100 N = 150 N.

39- A.   Zero

One AC cycle beginning at a current of zero amps and increasing will be complete after the current reaches its peak current in one direction, then decreases to zero then begins to flow in the opposite direction, increasing from a current of zero until it reaches the same peak current magnitude, then decreases back to zero. This cycle repeats 60 times per second. If there are 60 cycles/second, then in 1/120th of a second, (60 cycles/second)/(1/125 seconds) = 0.5 cycles. This is exactly one half to the AC cycle. At the half cycle, the current will have increased from zero amps to a peak amplitude and then decreased back to a current value of zero amps.

40- D.   200 watts

The power, or energy per second, that is dissipated as heat by the resistors in a circuit is given by the formula P = (V)(I), where I is the circuit current and V is the voltage of the circuit. This gives a solution of P = (20 V)(10 A) = 200 V-A. For electrical circuits, one V-A or volt-amp is equivalent to one watt of electrical power. So 200 V-A is therefore equal to 200 watts.

41- D.   Products and covalent compounds

The chemical reaction indicates that the substances on the left side of the arrow react to form the substances on the right side of the arrow. The left side substances CH_4 and O_2 are reactants and the right side substances H_2O and CO_2 are products. Both products are covalent compounds because carbon and oxygen prefer to complete their valence electron shells by sharing electrons with other atoms in the form of covalent bonds.

42- D.   A physical separation based on mass

Isotopes of an element have identical chemical reactivity, so no chemical process is likely to be able to separate isotopes of the same element. Isotopes also have nearly identical freezing points, so separation based on freezing points is also an ineffective approach. The mass of H^2 is twice that of H^1 so this is the most likely of the four methods to achieve a separation of the two isotopes.

43- D. Less than 1%

The hydrogen ion concentration of a solution with pH 3.7 is between 1×10^{-3} and 1×10^{-4} moles per liter. The pH of water is 7, which is equivalent to a hydrogen ion concentration of 1×10^{-7} moles per liter. This hydrogen ion concentration is 1000 times lower than the lower limit of the solutions hydrogen ion concentration; therefore, water is contributing at most 0.1% of the hydrogen ions in the solution.

44- B. Ribosomes

Ribosomes are the organelles that read messenger RNA and assemble the proteins that are encoded for in the messenger RNA. Viruses infecting a cell also must use ribosomes in a similar fashion to construct copies of their proteins.

45- D. There would be no tides on Earth that occur due to the effects of the moon

If the moon completed one orbit of the Earth in exactly the same amount of time that the Earth requires to complete one full rotation on its axis, then the moon would remain in a fixed position above the Earth. This would prevent the moon from exerting a changing gravitational force on the oceans. As a result, there would be no tides created by the gravitational influence of the moon.

46- B. Cartilage

Cartilage protects the ends of bones from mechanical injury at movable joints. Osteoarthritis is a common medical condition in the elderly that is the result of the loss of this protective cartilage.

47- C. Protection of the airway

The epiglottis is a hinge-like structure located in the throat at the entry point to the trachea, which is the beginning of the lower airway. When drinking or swallowing, the epiglottis closes over the top of the trachea and prevents solid or liquid material from either entering the trachea and possibly obstructing the flow of air or else passing to the lungs, resulting in lung damage or infection.

48- B. Pharynx

During inhalation, air first passes from the nasal cavity directly to the pharynx, then to the trachea, which contains the larynx, then to the primary bronchi, then to smaller bronchial branches and eventually to the alveoli in the lungs.

49- D. Oxygenated blood to the left atrium

The pulmonary vein is unique among veins in general, in that it is the only vein that transports oxygenated blood. It is classified as a vein because, by definition, any vessel carrying blood to the heart is a vein.

50- D. Receive blood from a person whose blood type is O positive

Blood types are based on molecules found on the surface of red blood cells. A, B and Rh factor are different surface molecules. Persons with "A" molecules are blood type A, those with "B" are blood type B, those with both A and B are blood type AB and those with neither A nor B are blood type O. If a person has Rh factor, they are blood type positive, and those without Rh factor are blood type negative. Persons may not receive blood with an A, B or Rh if they do not possess A, B or Rh as part of their blood type. A person with type A positive blood may receive blood from a person with type O blood for two reasons. The first is that type O does not have type B molecules on red blood cells. Type A blood cannot receive type B blood or type AB blood because both have B molecules. The second reason is that type O positive does have Rh molecules, but type A positive also has Rh molecules, so this is a compatible blood type for transfusion. Note that the reverse is not true. The type O positive donor cannot receive blood from the type A positive person.

51- B.   Emulsify fat
Bile is secreted from the gallbladder into the small intestines in order to emulsify or break large globs of fat into much smaller fat droplets so that the fat may be more easily absorbed through the walls of the intestine and into the bloodstream.

52- C.   Uterus
The endometrial lining of the uterus responds to hormones secreted during the menstrual cycle. It grows thicker at the beginning of the cycle and is shed as menstrual flow at the end of the cycle. During ovulation, the lining is at its thickest and most well-vascularized state, making it an ideal site for the implantation of a fertilized ovum.

53- A.   Coordination of movements
Precise and delicate movements require a tremendous amount of neural processing. This occurs primarily in the cerebellum. Visual processing occurs throughout the cerebral cortex, mostly in the occipital lobes. Simple reflexes like those described in choice C are routed through the spinal cord. Control of breathing and heartrate occurs in the medulla oblongata.

54- D.   The influenza agent is much less biologically complex than the strep throat agent
The infectious agent of influenza is a virus. It is much simpler biologically than a living cell such as the bacterium Streptococcus pyogenes, the infectious agent of strep throat. Viruses are not susceptible to antibiotics, but bacteria are. Neither viruses nor bacteria possess a nucleus.

55- A.   Cystic fibrosis
The cystic fibrosis gene is a mutation of a normal allele. A person must have both copies of the allele to develop the disease. Therefore, to develop the disease, one must receive one allele from both the person's mother and father. Huntington's disease is a dominant heritable disease, meaning that it requires only one copy of the gene in order to develop the disease. Mesothelioma is a cancer of the lining of the lung that is almost always associated with asbestos exposure. Tuberculosis is caused by a bacterium.

56- C.   Golgi apparatus
The Golgi apparatus packages substances synthesized by the cell into membrane-bound vesicles. The vesicles, along with their contents, are transported to the exterior cell membrane. The vesicles fuse with the membrane and empty their contents into the environment immediately outside of the cell.

57- C.   Occurs during both mitosis and meiosis

During cell division, the DNA of chromosomes is copied and stored as one of the two chromatids of the chromosomes. During anaphase of mitosis and meiosis 2, the sister chromatids are pulled apart to opposite poles of the cell and the cell begins to divide into two daughter cells.

58- A.   Autotrophs

Only autotrophs are capable of beginning a food web because they do not require the products of any other living organism in order to grow. They can then serve as the base of a chain that can include herbivores and then carnivores and omnivores. Note that herbivores, carnivores and omnivores are not required in a food web. A self-sustaining food web also requires decomposers. This simple food web of autotrophs in the form of plants and decomposer organisms was the only food web found on land for millions of years.

59- C.   Sedimentary to metamorphic

Throughout the Earth, within the upper two miles of crust, sedimentary rock is currently experiencing sufficient pressure from overlying material to cause the transformation process to metamorphic rock to proceed. Sedimentary and metamorphic rock can be drawn much deeper than two miles down into the Earth's interior and remelted into magma. This magma can form igneous rock, but this is a two-step process – melting and then cooling – so it is indirect, and part of the processes occurs much deeper than two miles from the Earth's surface.

60- C.   Carbon dioxide

The percentage composition of the Earth's atmosphere is: nitrogen 78%, oxygen 21%, argon 0.9% and carbon dioxide and other trace gases less than 0.1%

61- C.   One million watts

Power is the amount of work performed per unit time. The amount of work required to lift an object a certain height above the surface of the Earth is equal to the acceleration due to gravity, 10 m/s times the height above the surface of the Earth, 1000 m (1 kilometer) times the mass of the object; this is $(10,000 \text{ kg})(1000 \text{ m})(10 \text{ m/s}^2) = 10^8 \text{ J}$ (joules). Divide this by the time required to reach the maximum height, $10^8 \text{ J}/100 \text{ s } 10^\wedge$ or one million Watts.

62- D.   Located on separate chromosomes of a chromosome pair

The law of independent assortment occurs when two alleles of a gene each have an equal chance of being passed to an organism's offspring. Alleles of a gene almost never are located on different chromosome pairs. If the alleles are located on separate chromosomes of a chromosome pair, they are most likely to be separated into two gamete cells during meiosis. Thus each allele will have an equal chance of being passed to the male's offspring.

63- A.   Zero

If an object has a constant velocity, then the sum of all forces acting on the object or the net force must be zero. Any net force acting on an object will result in an acceleration of the object based on the formula $F_{net} = ma$. By definition, an object that is accelerating must be changing its velocity.

64- B.   1 gram of glucose

Glycogen is a large polymer molecule composed only of glucose molecules. It can be easily broken down into glucose molecules. This breakdown reaction of glycogen requires little if any energy and 1 gram of glycogen will break down into 1 gram of glucose. Therefore, the energy available to the body from glycogen is nearly identical to an equivalent mass of glucose.

65- C.   Decreases in direct proportion to the distance squared

Light emitted by a source can be thought of as concentric spherical shells of photons moving away from the source. Since the number of photons in any shell remains constant as the shell expands, its surface area increases as given by the formula for the area of a sphere, $A_s = \pi r^2$. As the radius, or distance, from the light source increases, the surface area of the photon shell increases proportionally to the square of the distance. Since the intensity of the light is the density of photons per unit area, the intensity of the light will also decrease in direct proportion to the distance squared.

66- D.   Noble gases

The group VIII elements have completely filled valence electron shells and therefore are the most chemically nonreactive of all the elements. This disdain for engaging in interactions with other elements is a somewhat humorous reference to the perception that in royal societies the noble classes did not associate with the lower classes.

67- B.   Velocity always increases

An object's kinetic energy is proportional to the square of its velocity. The mass of an object will actually increase with increasing velocity. It is possible that high velocities might increase an object's density, but most solids and liquids are incompressible, so usually their densities will not increase.

68- B.   Increased boiling point

Hydrogen bonding increases the attraction of individual molecules to each other. This means that it requires more energy in the form of heat to transition from lower to higher energy phases of matter. Boiling represents a transition from a lower matter phase, liquid, to a higher energy phase, gas. Therefore, this transition will occur at a higher temperature if the individual molecules are hydrogen bonding with each other.

69- A.   At the border region of colliding warm and cold fronts

The collision of a warm front and a cold front results in the strong updrafts of warm air through cold air. This is the process that is most favorable to the production of the largest and most extensive cumulous clouds among the choices above.

70- B.   Because the Earth is in orbit around the sun

If the Earth did not orbit the sun, the moon would cross between the Earth and sun once for every moon orbit of the Earth. Because the Earth is constantly changing its angular position relative to the sun, the moon will find itself between the sun and the moon less often than once per lunar month.

71- C.   Endocrine glands

The ovaries synthesize and release the hormone estrogen into the bloodstream. Any tissue or organ that synthesizes and releases hormones into the bloodstream is, by definition, an endocrine gland.

72- A. There are no omnivores that are also autotrophs

No animals are autotrophs and no plants, which are autotrophs, also consume both meat and other plants. Carnivores usually also eat plant matter, so they are technically omnivores, carnivores are frequently scavengers, or consumers of dead animals which they did not kill themselves. A detritivore eats tiny bits of organic matter, so by definition detritivores are also scavengers.

73- C. By decreasing convective and conductive heat loss only

Since the vacuum gap separates the inner container surface from the outer container surface, both conductive and convective heat loss is isolated from the outer surface of the container. Radiative heat loss can occur through a vacuum, so this method is relatively ineffective at limiting this form of heat loss.

74- D. She can pull both herself and the basket upward toward the horizontal bar if the basket weighs less than 60 kg

If the basket weighs more than the woman, the woman will begin to lift herself off of the surface of the basket when she exerts a pulling force on the rope that exceeds the force of gravity acting on her. At this point, she will not be able to exert any greater pulling force. If the basket weighs less than the woman, the basket will begin to exert an upward force on the woman's feet before she is able to pull herself off of the surface of the basket. With additional pulling force, both the basket and the woman will lift upward together.

75- A. Volcanic eruptions

Carbon that has always existed deep in the interior of the Earth can be converted to carbon dioxide by geological processes and emitted into the Earth's atmosphere during volcanic eruptions; this process generates new carbon dioxide. Hydroelectric power does not generate any carbon dioxide. Even if boron underwent radioactive decay, that process would result in decay to elements with atomic numbers lower than boron's atomic number; carbon's atomic number is larger than boron's atomic number. The use of fossil fuels does not generate carbon that did not previously exist as carbon dioxide in the Earth's atmosphere. Fossil fuels are products of previously living organisms. All of the carbon in living organisms originates from carbon dioxide that is absorbed by plants from the Earth's atmosphere.

76- C. Facilitation of bowel movements

Dietary fiber adds bulk to fecal material, which aids in the passage of the material out of the body. This leads to easier and more regular bowel movements. Lack of dietary fiber has been shown to be associated with increased risk for colon cancer.

77- B. The Earth's outer core

Molten iron in the Earth's outer core generates the Earth's magnetic field. Without circulating ferromagnetic material in the Earth's interior, the Earth's magnetic field would be nearly nonexistent. This is the case with the planet Mars, whose liquid core apparently solidified billions of years ago. This left Mars unprotected from the pressure of the solar wind, leading to the loss of almost the entirety of Mars' atmosphere.

78- A.   The Precambrian eon

Although microscopic and a few macroscopic fossils do exist that predate the end of the Precambrian eon, the end of the eon is marked by an explosive increase in the numbers of macroscopic fossils in the geological record.

79- B.   P orbitals

P orbitals are bi-lobed or dumbbell shaped. When two p orbitals are in close proximity, their upper lobes and their lower lobes can overlap and reconfigure into a bi-lobed hybrid bonding orbital called a pi bond. None of the other orbitals mentioned in the answer choices above are able to form pi bonds.

80- A.   The gravitational constant g

The force of gravity can vary, but the constant g for the universal force of gravity is the same everywhere in the universe. There is an upper limit to the speed of light, but the speed of light changes when light passes through materials with different indices of refraction. The mass of a proton is the same everywhere in the universe, but the weight of a proton depends on the strength of its local gravitational field. The size of the universe has expanded, and continues to expand, since the big bang. In fact, scientists have found that the expansion of the universe is actually accelerating. No new matter is entering the universe, so the matter density of the universe is decreasing as the volume of the universe continues to increase.

81- B.   Low-pressure systems

Extreme low-pressure systems that are moving across large areas of open water such as oceans and seas, with very warm surface water temperatures, can generate the largest, most powerful and most destructive storms on Earth. Depending on the hemisphere in which they occur, these storms are called hurricanes, cyclones or typhoons.

82- B.   Oort cloud, asteroid belt and Kuiper belt

The Van Allen belt is a region of high radiation that encircles the Earth. The Magellanic cloud is actually a satellite galaxy of our home galaxy, the Milky Way. Proxima Centauri is the nearest star to our sun.

83- C.   A total number of 23 unpaired chromosomes

The diploid or somatic human cell contains 23 pairs of chromosomes, 22 pairs of autosomes and one set of sex chromosomes, which can be an X and a Y chromosome or two X chromosomes. The human gametes, sperm and ova, are haploid, meaning they contain one half of the normal number of chromosomes as a human diploid cell. The gamete has one copy of each of the 22 autosomes and one sex chromosome, either X or Y, for a total number of 23 chromosomes.

84- C.   A collection of all interdependent species in a geographical region

For answer choice A, there may be more than one ecological community that shares the same geographical region. Ecological communities always consist of more than one species. The other answer choices are defined as comprising only one species.

85- C.   The amino acids that are only available through dietary intake

The essential amino acids cannot be synthesized by the body. The only source of these amino acids is from dietary intake.

86- B.   A slower axial rotation

It is somewhat surprising that Saturn, which is vastly larger and more massive than the Earth, has a significantly shorter rotational period than the Earth and is remarkably less dense than the Earth. Saturn is much farther away from the sun, so its orbital radius is much larger than the Earth. Saturn's magnetic field is much stronger than the Earth's magnetic field.

87- A.   Pepsin

One is not expected to know all of the substances secreted by various bodily organs, but pepsin is the major substance besides hydrochloric acid that is secreted by the stomach, and this is expected knowledge for the exam.

88- C.   Osteoporosis (bone demineralization)

Vitamin D is required to absorb calcium from one's diet. Vitamin D deficiency over time will result in inadequate calcium intake. Bone is composed of a mineral (hydroxyapatite) that has a high calcium content. Calcium is also required in significant amounts by every cell in the body. With inadequate calcium levels, the body will begin to break bone down to extract the bone calcium (demineralization for use elsewhere in the body. This will lead to loss of bone density and weakening of the mechanical strength of the bones. This disease process is known as osteoporosis.

89- A.   The elevator is accelerating downward at 4.9 m/s^2

For the man's apparent weight to decrease by 50%, the net acceleration downward must be exactly half of the acceleration due to gravity. This would result in a downward acceleration of g/2. The acceleration of gravity at or near the surface of the Earth is 9.8 m/s^2. One half of this value is 4.9 m/s^2. The exam will probably provide the numerical value for g, but this is basic information that is expected to be known by those taking the exam. The elevator is actually exerting an upward force equal to exactly half of the downward force due to gravity. This gives a net force on the scale equal to half of the net force on the scale when the elevator is motionless.

90- C.   Positrons

Positrons are identical to electrons with the exception that they have a positive rather than a negative electric charge. Protons are identical to anti-protons except for having opposite charges. An atom with antiprotons in its nucleus, orbited by an equal number of electrically bound positrons, would be a neutral atom. This type of atom is an example of anti-matter and antimatter has been proven to exist.

91- A.   Radio waves

Since all forms of electromagnetic energy, including visible light, are energy waves, they will be subject to the Doppler effect. Visible light detected from a source that is receding from the detector will be stretched out, resulting in an increase in the wavelength of the light. Ultraviolet light, X-rays and gamma rays all have shorter wavelengths than visible light. Among the choices above, only radio waves have longer wavelengths compared to the wavelengths of visible light. If the galaxy is receding at a high enough velocity, visible light emitted from the galaxy could be stretched out to the length of radio waves as they reach the Earth.

92- A.   The two pieces will each have a positive and negative magnetic pole

In natural magnets, the atoms of the magnet are all aligned in the same direction with respect to the spin of their lone unpaired valence electrons. No matter how such a magnet is cut into pieces, each piece will retain this alignment of atoms; therefore every piece itself will be an individual magnet with both a positive and negative magnetic pole.

93- B.   Coelenterata

Although there are thousands of biological subclassifications, one should be aware that in the kingdom Plantae (plants), the four major phyla, which are immediately below the kingdom level, are Bryophyta, Tracheophyta, Gymnospermia and angiospermia. Coelenterates are animals.

94- C.   Potassium (K) atom to a sulfur (S) atom

If an atom of a given element loses three protons from its nucleus, it will become an atom of an element that has an atomic number that is three less than the original atom's elemental atomic number. Among the choice pairs above, only potassium, with an atomic number of 19, and sulfur, with an atomic number of 16, differ by an atomic number of three.

95- A.   Magnesium and chlorine

Magnesium is in the alkali Earth or group II column on the periodic table. Group II elements have two valence electrons and form ionic salt crystal compounds with highly electronegative elements, in particular, the group VII or halide elements, which include chlorine, fluorine and bromine. The halides require one additional electron to complete their valence shells. Group II elements lose both valence electrons to group VII elements in ionic compounds and are therefore +2 atomic ions. Since a group VII element will accept only one electron per atom, two group VII atoms are required to accept the two electrons from each group II atom in an ionic crystalline compound. This requires that the compound contain two group VII atoms for each group II atom. Lithium and sodium are group I elements and have only one valence electron per atom, These elements will form one-to-one ratio ionic crystal compounds with the group VII elements. Oxygen is a group VI element and requires two electrons to complete its valence shell. In a compound with calcium, a group II element, the ratio of calcium to oxygen will be one to one.

96- C.   Adjacent to and above the stratosphere

Beginning at the surface of the Earth, the layers of the atmosphere are the troposphere, stratosphere, ozone layer, mesosphere and the thermosphere.

97- D.   A high HDL level and low LDL level

HDL (high-density lipoprotein) cholesterol is considered to be "good" cholesterol. Higher levels are associated with lower levels of cholesterol-related disease processes. LDL (low-density lipoprotein) cholesterol is considered to be "bad" cholesterol and high levels are associated with increased cholesterol-related disease processes. In humans, for any age range, the ideal cholesterol profile is a high HDL level and low LDL level. This is also referred to as a high HDL-to-LDL cholesterol ratio.

98- B.   A one-degree increase on the Fahrenheit scale is a smaller temperature increase than a one-degree increase on the Celsius scale

The relative size of the temperature increase for the two temperature scales can be determined by comparing the range between the freezing and boiling points of water. On the Fahrenheit scale, this is 32 degrees to 212 degrees. On the Celsius scale, this is zero degrees to 100 degrees. Clearly there are more Fahrenheit degrees between this water freezing point – boiling point range than Celsius degrees, therefore a one-degree Fahrenheit temperature change represents a smaller absolute incremental change in temperature than does a one-degree Celsius temperature change.

99- C.   As a liquid, from the Earth's surface, to underground reservoirs

Infiltration is the term used to describe the process in the water cycle where water in the liquid phase that is at the ground surface filters through the underlying soil and porous earthen layers until it reaches an underground collecting reservoir. This is the process that creates the subsurface "water table" that often serves as a source of water for drinking and irrigation. These reservoirs can be gigantic, as is the case with the Ogallala Aquifer, which provides most of the irrigation water for the vast farming regions of the Central Plains of the United States.

100-   B.   Shares the same climate

A biome is large community of plants and animals that occupies a distinct contiguous geographical region that has the same climate and dominant plant species. Examples of biomes are grassland, desert and tropical rainforest.

INTERMEDIATE PRACTICE TEST: MATHEMATICS

1 – C. 12%

To find the percent increase, you first need to know the amount of the increase. Enrollment went from 3,450 in 2010 to 3,864 in 2015. This is an increase of 414. Now, to find the percent of the increase, divide the amount of the increase by the original amount:

$$414 \div 3,450 = 0.12$$

To convert a decimal to a percent, move the decimal point two places to the right:
$$0.12 = 12\%$$

When a question asks for the percent increase or decrease, divide the amount of the increase or decrease by the original amount.

2 – C. 78

To find the median in a series of numbers, arrange the numbers in order from smallest to largest:

$$69, 73, 78, 80, 100$$

The number in the center is the median. If there are an even number of numbers in the series, for example:

34, 46, 52, 54, 67, 81

then the median will be the average of the two numbers in the center. In this example, the median will be 53 (the average of 52 and 54). Remember: the median is not the same as the average.

3 – D. 22

This question asks you to find the square root of 11 times 44. First, do the multiplication: 11 * 44 = 484. Now multiply each of the possible answers by itself to see which one is the square root of 484.

4 – A. 16 gallons

Amy drives her car until the gas tank is 1/8 full. This means that it is 7/8 empty. She fills it by adding 14 gallons. In other words, 14 gallons is 7/8 of the tank's capacity. Draw a simple diagram to represent the gas tank.

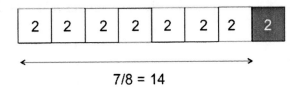

7/8 = 14

You can see that each eighth of the tank is 2 gallons. So the capacity of the tank is 2 * 8, or 16.

5 – D. 3^4

Positive numbers are larger than negative numbers, so this limits the possible answers to 42 and 3^4. 3^4 equals 81 (3 * 3 * 3 * 3).

6 – C. 59

A prime number is a whole number greater than 1 that can be divided evenly only by itself and 1. In this question, only 59 fits that definition. 81 is not prime because it can be divided evenly by 9; 49 is not prime because it can be divided evenly by 7; and 77 is not prime because it can be divided evenly by 7 and 11.

7 – D. $\dfrac{(6)(9)}{2}$

The area of a triangle is one-half the product of the base and the height. Choices A and B are incorrect because they add the base and the height instead of multiplying them. Choice C is incorrect because it multiplies the product of the base and the height by 2 instead of dividing it by 2.

8 – A. 2,595

The steps in evaluating a mathematical expression must be carried out in a certain order, which is called "the order of operations." These are the steps in order:

Parentheses: The first step is to do any operations in parentheses.
Exponents: Then do any steps that involve exponents.

Multiply and Divide: Multiply and divide from left to right.
Add and Subtract: Add and subtract from left to right.

One way to remember this order is to use this sentence:
Please **E**xcuse **M**y **D**ear **A**unt **S**ally.

To evaluate the expression in this question, follow these steps:

Multiply the numbers in **Parentheses**: 3 * 4 = 12
Apply the **Exponent** 2 to the number in parentheses: $12^2 = 144$
Multiply: 6 * 3 * 144 = 2,592
Add: 2 + 2,592 + 1 = 2,595

---

9 – B. 9

The symbol $\geq$ means "greater than or equal to." The only answer that is greater than or equal to 9 is 9.

---

10 – C. 81

When two numbers with the same sign (both positive or both negative) are multiplied, the answer is a positive number. When two numbers with different signs (one positive and the other negative) are multiplied, the answer is negative.

---

11 – B. $x = a^5$

When multiplying numbers that have the same base and different exponents, keep the base the same and add the exponents. In this case, $a^2 * a^3$ becomes $a^{(2+3)}$ or a^5.

---

12 – C. $310

The costs of all these items can be expressed in terms of the cost of the ream of paper. Use x to represent the cost of a ream of paper. The flash drive costs three times as much as the ream of paper, so it costs $3x$. The textbook costs three times as much as the flash drive, so it costs $9x$. The printer cartridge costs twice as much as the textbook, so it costs $18x$. So now we have:

$$x + 3x + 9x + 18x = 31x$$

The ream of paper costs $10, so $31x$ (the total cost) is $310.

---

13 – C. 6

Solve the equation:

$$x > 3^2 - 4$$
$$x > 9 - 4$$
$$x > 5$$

We know that x is greater than 5, so the answer could be either 6 or 7. The question asks for the smallest possible value of x, so the correct answer is 6.

14 –   A. 84

First, find the number of girls in the class. Convert 52% to a decimal by moving the decimal point two places to the left:

$$52\% = .52$$

Now, multiply .52 times the number of students in the class:

$$.52 * 350 = 182$$

Of the 182 girls, 98 plan to go to college, so 84 do not plan to go to college.

$$182 - 98 = 84$$

---

15 –   C. $300

If the phone was on sale at 30% off, the sale price was 70% of the original price. So

$$\$210 = 70\% \text{ of } x$$

where x is the original price of the phone. When you convert 70% to a decimal, you get:

$$\$210 = .70 * x$$

To isolate x on one side of the equation, divide both sides of the equation by .70. You find that $x =$ $300.

---

16 –   A. 10

Use the facts you are given to write an equation:
$$7 + 4/5n = 15$$

First, subtract 7 from both sides of the equation. You get:
$$4/5n = 8$$
Now divide both sides of the equation by 4/5. To divide by a fraction, invert the fraction (4/5 becomes 5/4) and multiply:

$$n = \frac{8}{1} * \frac{5}{4}$$
$$n = \frac{40}{4}$$
$$n = 10$$

---

17 –   D. 108

The ratio of the two numbers is 7:3. This means that the larger number is 7/10 of 360 and the smaller number is 3/10 of 360.

$$\frac{3}{10} * \frac{360}{1} = \frac{1,080}{10} = 108$$

---

18 –   A. 20

Alicia must have a score of 75% on a test with 80 questions. To find how many questions she must answer correctly, first convert 75% to a decimal by moving the decimal point two places to the left: 75% = .75. Now multiply .75 times 80:

$$.75 * 80 = 60.$$

Alicia must answer 60 questions correctly, but the question asks how many questions can she miss. If she must answer 60 correctly, then she can miss 20.

---

19 –   B. 3,024 cubic inches

The formula for the volume of a rectangular solid is length * width * height. So the volume of this box is:

$$18 * 12 * 14 = 3,024 \text{ cubic inches}$$

---

20 –   B. Perpendicular

Lines that form a right angle are called perpendicular.

---

21 –   C. 15 square feet

This shape is called a parallelogram. The area of a parallelogram equals the base times the height.

---

22 –   D. 0.72

The simplest way to answer this question is to convert the fractions to decimals. To convert a fraction to a decimal, divide the numerator (the top number) by the denominator (the bottom number).

$$5/8 = 0.625$$
$$3/5 = 0.6$$
$$2/3 = 0.67$$

The largest number is 0.72.

---

23 –   A. 11

If Charles wrote an average of 7 pages per day for four days, he wrote a total of 28 pages. He wrote a total of 17 pages on the first three days, so he must have written 11 pages on the fourth day.

---

24 –   B. 3.44 square feet

Find the area of the square by multiplying the length of a side by itself. The area of the square is 16 square feet. Now find the area of the circle by using this formula:

$$A = \pi r^2$$

The symbol π equals approximately 3.14. The letter r is the radius of the circle. In this case, r is half the width of the square (or 2), so r^2 is 4. Therefore, the area of the circle is

$$A = 3.14 * 4$$
$$A = 12.56$$

To find the area of the square that is not covered by the circle, subtract 12.56 square feet from 16 square feet.

---

25 – B. $\dfrac{20}{mp^2}$

To divide by a fraction, invert the second fraction and multiply.

So $\dfrac{5}{mp} \div \dfrac{p}{4}$ becomes $\dfrac{5}{mp} * \dfrac{4}{p}$

$$\dfrac{5}{mp} * \dfrac{4}{p} = \dfrac{20}{mp^2}$$

---

26 – B. 10 miles

If you made a simple map with these three cities, it would look like this:

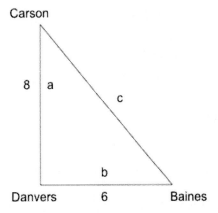

This is a right triangle. The longest side of a right triangle is called the hypotenuse. The two legs of the triangle are labeled *a* and *b*. The hypotenuse is labeled *c*. You can find the length of the hypotenuse (the distance between Caron and Baines) by using this equation:

$$a^2 + b^2 = c^2$$

In this case, the equation would be:

$$8^2 + 6^2 = c^2$$

$$or$$

$$64 + 36 = c^2$$

$$100 = c^2$$

To find *c*, ask yourself: What number times itself equals 100? The answer is 10.

---

27 – C. 3/36

When you roll a pair of 6-sided dice, there are 36 possible combinations of numbers (or outcomes) that can result. There are six numbers on each of the dice, so there are 6 * 6 possible combinations. Only three of those combinations will yield a total of 10: 4+6, 5+5, and 6+4. Much of the time, probability answers will be given in the form of simplified fractions. In this case, the correct answer could also have been 1/12.

---

28 – A. $144

When one person dropped out of the arrangement, the cost for the remaining three went up by $12 per person for a total of $36. This means that each person's share was originally $36. There were four people in the original arrangement, so the cost of the gift was 4 * $36, or $144.

Or alternatively:

Let 4x equal the original cost of the gift. If the number of shares decreases to 3, then the total cost is 3(x+12). Those expressions must be equal, so:

$$4x = 3(x+12)$$
$$4x = 3x + 36$$

Subtracting 3x from both sides, we get:

$$x = 36$$

Then the original price of the gift was 4 times 36, or $144.

---

29 – C. 120

The factorial of a number is the product of all the integers less than or equal to the number. The factorial of 5 is 5 * 4 * 3 * 2 * 1 = 120. The factorial is written this way: 5!

---

30 – D. 7

In this number:

1 is in the thousands place.
2 is in the hundreds place.
3 is in the tens place.
4 is in the ones place

---

5 is in the tenths place.

6 is in the hundredths place.

7 is in the thousandths place.

---

31 – B. 4

The mode is the number that appears most often in a set of numbers.

Since 4 appears three times, it is the "Mode."

---

32 – C. 49

A perfect square is the product of an integer times itself. In this question, 49 is a perfect square because it is the product of 7 and 7.

---

33 – A. (14 + 24) * 8 * 5

In the correct answer, (14 + 24) * 8 * 5, the hourly wages of Amanda and Oscar are first combined, and then this amount is multiplied by 8 hours in a day and five days in a week. One of the other choices, 14 + 24 * 8 * 5, looks similar to this, but it is incorrect because the hourly wages must be combined before they can be multiplied by 8 and 5.

---

34 – D. 130,500

The population of Mariposa County in 2015 was 90% of its population in 2010. Convert 90% to a decimal by moving the decimal point two places to the left: 90% = .90. Now multiply .90 times 145,000 (the population in 2010).

$$.90 * 145,000 = 130,500$$

---

35 – C. 17/24

To add 1/3 and 3/8, you must find a common denominator. The simplest way to do this is to multiply the denominators: 3 * 8 = 24. Therefore, 24 is a common denominator. (This method will not always give you the <u>lowest</u> common denominator, but it does in this case.)

Once you have found a common denominator, you need to convert both fractions in the problem to equivalent fractions that have that same denominator. To do this, multiply each fraction by an equivalent of 1.

$$\frac{1}{3} * \frac{8}{8} = \frac{8}{24}$$

$$\frac{3}{8} * \frac{3}{3} = \frac{9}{24}$$

Now you can add 8/24 and 9/24 to solve the problem.

---

36 – B. Serena is 7, Tom is 4

Use S to represent Serena's age. Tom is 3 years younger than Serena, so his age is S–3. In 4 years, Tom will be twice as old as Serena was 3 years ago. So you can write this equation:

$$\text{Tom} + 4 = 2(\text{Serena} - 3)$$

Now substitute S for Serena and S–3 for Tom.

$$(S - 3) + 4 = 2(S - 3)$$

Simplify the equation.

$$S + 1 = 2S - 6$$

Subtract S from both sides of the equation. You get:

$$1 = S - 6$$

Add 6 to both sides of the equation. You get:

$$7 = S, \text{ Serena's age}$$

$$4 = S - 3, \text{ Tom's age}$$

---

37 –   A. Length = 12, width = 4

Use w to represent the width of the rectangle. The length is three times the width, so the length is $3w$. The area of the rectangle is the length times the width, so the area is $w * 3w$, or $3w^2$.

$$3w^2 = 48$$

Divide both sides of the equation by 3. You get:

$$w^2 = 16$$

$$w = 4, \text{ the width of the rectangle}$$
$$3w = 12, \text{ the length of the rectangle}$$

---

38 –   B. 24 = 2 * 2 * 2 * 3

The prime factors of a number are the prime numbers that divide that number evenly. The prime factorization of a number is a list of the prime factors that must be multiplied to yield that number.

The simplest method of finding the prime factorization is to start with a simple multiplication fact for that number. In this case, we could have chosen:

$$24 = 6 * 4$$

The prime factorization of 24 includes the prime factorization of both 6 and 4. Since 6 = 2 * 3 and 4 = 2 * 2, the prime factorization of 24 must be:

$$24 = 2 * 2 * 2 * 3$$

39 –   A. A number greater than x

When a positive number is divided by a positive number less than 1, the quotient will always be larger than the number being divided. For example, 5 ÷ 0.5 = 10. If we solve this as a fraction, 5 ÷ (1/2) is the same as 5 * (2/1), which equals 10, since dividing by a fraction is the same as multiplying by the reciprocal.

40 –   C. x = 11

Subtracting a negative number is the same as adding a positive number. So 8 – (–3) is the same as 8 + 3, which equals 11.

41 –   C. The square of a number is always a positive number.

When two numbers with the same sign (positive or negative) are multiplied, the product is always positive. When a number is squared, it is multiplied by itself, so the numbers being multiplied have the same sign. Therefore, the product is always positive.

The square of a number greater than 1 is always greater than the number. But the square of a positive number less than one (for example 0.5) is always less than the original number.

42 –   B. 515

Marisol scored higher than 78% of the students who took the test. Convert 78% to a decimal by moving the decimal point two places to the left: 78% = .78. Now multiply .78 times the number of students who took the test:

$$.78 * 660 = 514.8 \text{ or } 515 \text{ students (must be whole numbers)}$$

43 –   D. $12

Use the information given to write an equation:

$$530 = 40d + 50$$

When you subtract 50 from both sides of the equation, you get:

$$480 = 40d$$

Divide both sides of the equation by 40.

$$12 = d, \text{ Sam's hourly wage}$$

44 –   **D.** $r = \dfrac{p-3}{2}$

Begin by subtracting 3 from both sides of the equation. You get:

$$p - 3 = 2r$$

Now, to isolate r on one side of the equation, divide both sides of the equation by 2. You get:

$$r = \dfrac{p-3}{2}$$

---

45 –   **B.** 40

The least common multiple is used when finding the lowest common denominator. The least common multiple is the lowest number that can be divided evenly by both of the numbers.

Here is a simple method to find the least common multiple of 8 and 10. Write 8 on the left side of your paper, then add 8 and write the result, then add another 8 to that number and write the result. Keep going until you have a list that looks something like this:

    8 16 24 32 40…

This is a partial list of multiples of 8. (If you remember your multiplication tables, these numbers are the column or row that go with 8.)

Now do the same thing with 10.

    10 20 30 40 …

This is the partial list of multiples of 10.

Eventually, similar numbers will appear in both rows. The smallest of these numbers is the least common multiple. There will always be more multiples that are found in both rows, but the smallest number is the least common multiple.

---

46 –   **D.** $x = 4$

When you multiply or divide numbers that have the same sign (both positive or both negative), the answer will be positive. When you multiply or divide numbers that have different signs (one positive and the other negative), the answer will be negative. In this case, both numbers have the same sign. Divide as you normally would, and remember that the answer will be a positive number.

47 – A. $2\dfrac{5}{6}$

To convert an improper fraction to a mixed number, divide the numerator by the denominator. In this case, you get 2 with a remainder of 5. 2 becomes the whole number portion of the mixed number, and 5 becomes the numerator of the fraction.

---

48 – B. –10

To find the value of q, divide both sides of the equation by –13. When a positive number is divided by a negative number, the answer is negative.

---

49 – A. 12

Replace the letters with the numbers they represent, then perform the necessary operations.

$$3^2 + 6(0.5)$$

$$9 + 3 = 12$$

---

50 – B. 32 inches

The radius of a circle is one-half the diameter, so the diameter of this circle is 8 inches. The diameter is a line that passes through the center of a circle and joins two points on its circumference. If you study this figure, you can see that the diameter of the circle is the same as the length of each side of the square. The diameter is 8 inches, so the perimeter of the square is 32 inches (8+ 8 + 8 + 8).

---

51 – D. 21/32

To multiply fractions, multiply the numerators and the denominators. In this case, multiply 3 by 7, and 4 by 8. The correct answer is 21/32.

---

52 – B. 500,000,000

A billion is 1,000 million (1,000,000,000). Half a billion is 500 million (500,000,000).

---

53 – D. $y = 2x + 7$

The simplest way to answer this question is to see which of the equations would work for all the values of x and y in the table.

Choices A and D would work when x = 0 and y = 7, but A would not work for any other values of x and y.

Choice B would work when x = 3 and y = 13, but it would not work for any other values of x and y.

Choice C would not work for any of the values of x and y.

Only choice D would be correct for each ordered pair in the table.

---

54 – D. 80

If we call the smaller number x, then the larger number is 5x. The sum of the two numbers is 480, so:

$$x + 5x = 480$$

$$6x = 480$$

$$x = 80$$

---

55 –   C. 20

To solve this problem, first convert 45% to a decimal by moving the decimal point two places to the left: 45% = .45. Use x to represent the total number of students in the class. Then:

$$.45x = 9$$

Solve for x by dividing both sides of the equation by .45. 9 divided by .45 is 20.

---

56 –   A. 64 ft

We know the dimensions of the left side and the top side of this figure, but how can we find the dimensions of the other sides? Look at the two horizontal lines on the bottom of the figure. We know that together they are as wide as the top side of the figure, so together they must be 18 ft. Now look at the two vertical lines on the right side of the figure. We know that together they are as tall as the left side of the figure, so together they must be 14 ft. So now we know that the perimeter of the figure is 14 + 18 + 14 + 18, or 32 + 32 = 64 ft.

---

57 –   C. 4

Make a list of the powers of 10.

$10^2 = 100$
$10^3 = 1,000$
$10^4 = 10,000$
$10^5 = 100,000$

When you divide 15,200 by 1.52, you get 10,000, so the correct exponent is 4.

That exponent is also the number of places the decimal must be moved in the number 1.52 to make the number 15,200.

---

58 –   B. 6.5 * 10^{-3}

 Make a list of the negative powers of 10:

$10^{-2} = 0.01$
$10^{-3} = 0.001$
$10^{-4} = 0.0001$

$10^{-5} = 0.00001$

Now multiply each of these numbers by 6.5 to see which one gives you 0.0065. The decimal must be moved 3 places to the left in the number 6.5 to make the number 0.0065.

---

59 –   B. 32 diet, 80 regular

If the owner sells 2 diet sodas for every 5 regular sodas, then 2/7 of the sodas sold are diet and 5/7 are regular. Multiply these fractions by the total number of sodas sold:

$$\frac{2}{7} * \frac{112}{1} = \frac{224}{7} = 32$$

$$\frac{5}{7} * \frac{112}{1} = \frac{560}{7} = 80$$

Remember: when multiplying a fraction by a whole number, it is usually simpler to divide by the denominator first, then multiply by the numerator.

---

60 –   C. 16

The greatest common factor of two numbers is the largest number that can be divided evenly into both numbers. The simplest way to answer this question is to start with the largest answer (32) and see if it can be divided evenly into 48 and 64. It can't. Now try the next largest answer (16), and you see that it can be divided evenly into 48 and 64. 16 is the correct answer. The other answers are also factors, but the largest of them is 16.

---

61 –   B. 4.5 inches

The length of the larger rectangle is 12 inches, and the length of the smaller rectangle is 8 inches. Therefore, the length of the larger rectangle is 1.5 times the length of the smaller rectangle. Since the rectangles are proportional, the width of the larger rectangle must be 1.5 times the width of the smaller rectangle.

$$1.5 * 3 \text{ inches} = 4.5 \text{ inches}$$

---

62 –   D. 150 pounds

The average weight of the five friends is 180 pounds, so the total weight of all five is 5 times 180 or 900 pounds. Add the weights of Al, Bob, Carl, and Dave. Together, they weigh 750 pounds. Subtract 750 from 900 to find Ed's weight of 150 pounds.

---

63 –   A. –116

Calculate the value of x^2 and y^3, then add the results.

$$x^2 = (-3)\,(-3) = 9$$

$$y^3 = (-5)\,(-5)\,(-5) = -125$$

$$9 + (-125) = -116$$

---

64 –   C. 15 miles

Rebecca's commute is shorter than Alan's but longer than Bob's. Alan's commute is 18 miles, and Bob's is 14 miles, so Rebecca's must be longer than 14 but shorter than 18. Neither 14 nor 18 is correct, since the distances cannot be equal to either of the examples. Therefore, 15 is the only correct answer.

---

65 –   A. 10%

First, find the total number of patients admitted to the ER by adding the number admitted for all the reasons given in the question. There were 120 patients admitted. To find what percent were admitted for respiratory problems, divide the number admitted for respiratory problems by the total number admitted:

$$12 \div 120 = .10$$

Convert this decimal to a percent by moving the decimal point two places to the right: .10 = 10%. When you are asked what percent of a total is a certain part, divide the part by the whole.

---

66 –   C. 16

There are 9 times as many female nurses as male nurses. To find the number of male nurses, divide the number of female nurses by 9 ($144 \div 9 = 16$).

---

67 –   D. 64

If you drew a diagram of the larger square, you would see that you can make 8 rows of 8 smaller squares, so you can make a total of 64 squares.

---

68 –   A. 2 is the only even prime number.

2 is the only even prime number because all other even numbers are multiples of 2.

The largest prime number less than 100 is 97, not 89.

The greatest common factor of 24 and 42 is 6. The greatest common factor of two numbers is the largest number that can be divided evenly <u>into</u> both numbers.

The least common multiple of 8 and 6 is 24. The least common multiple of two numbers is the smallest number that can be divided evenly <u>by</u> both numbers.

---

69 –   C. 7/10

The simplest way to solve this problem is to convert the fractions to decimals. You do this by dividing the numerators by the denominators.

$2/3 = 0.67$ and $3/4 = 0.75$, so the correct answer is a decimal that falls between these two numbers.

$3/5 = 0.6$

$4/5 = 0.8$

$7/10 = 0.7$

$5/8 = 0.625$

---

70 –   A. 6

If $a = 10$, then $2a = 20$.

Now compute the value of b^2.

$$b^2 = (-b)(-b)$$
$$b^2 = (-4)(-4)$$
$$b^2 = 16$$

So, now you have:

$$\sqrt{20+16} \text{ or } \sqrt{36}$$

The square root of 36 is 6.

---

71 –   A. 1

The slope of a line is defined as "rise over run." You might also describe the slope of a line as the change in y over the change in x. You can see on this graph that the change in y over the change in x is 2/2, which is equal to 1. The slope of this line is positive because it is moving upward and increasing from left to right.

---

72 –   D. June

To find the median in a series of numbers, arrange the numbers in order from smallest to largest. The number in the center, 92 in this case, is the median.

---

73 –   B. 6

There are 3 state legislators on the committee, and these legislators make up 1/5 of its members. So there are a total of 15 members on the committee. Of these 15 members, 3 are state legislators and 6 are state employees, so 6 must be members of the public.

---

74 –   B. 1/5

After Mark chooses the first letter, there will be five letters remaining. So the probability that the second letter he chooses will be an M or an N is 1/5.

---

75 –   D. 3,105

The ratio of female to male students is exactly 5 to 4, so 5/9 of the students are female and 4/9 of the students are male. This means that the total number of students must be evenly divisible by 9, and 3,105 is the only answer that fits this requirement.

---

76 –   A. 0.6 * 90

To find 60% of 90, first convert 60% to a decimal by moving the decimal point two places to the left, then multiply this decimal (0.6) by 90.

77 –   C. 32 square inches

The perimeter of the rectangle is 24 inches. This means that the length plus the width must equal half of 24, or 12 inches. The ratio of length to width is 2:1, so the length is 2/3 of 12 and the width is 1/3 of 12. So the length is 8 inches and the width is 4 inches. The area (length times width) is 32 square inches.

78 –   B. The Bulldogs will definitely not be in the playoffs.

The Rangers are playing the Statesmen in the final game, so one of these teams will finish with a record of eleven wins and two losses. Even if the Bulldogs win their game, their final record will be ten wins and three losses. So the Bulldogs will not be in the playoffs.

79 –   A. 134,000

Make a list of the powers of 10.

$10^2 = 100$
$10^3 = 1,000$
$10^4 = 10,000$
$10^5 = 100,000$

When you multiply 1.34 by 100,000, you get 134,000.

80 –   B. –62

When you substitute 4 for a, you get:

$$(-4 * -4 * -4) - (-4) - 2$$

The product $(-4 * -4 * -4) = -64$. Subtracting (-4) is the same as adding 4.

So now you have:
$$-64 + 4 - 2 = -62$$

81 –   A. $52,000

Convert 15% to a decimal by moving the decimal point two places to the left: 15% = 0.15. Using x to represent Brian's gross salary, you can write this equation:

$$0.15x = \$7,800$$

To solve for x, divide both sides of the equation by 0.15. $7,800 divided by 0.15 is $52,000.

82 –   C. $3^3 * 5 * 2$

For each of the answers, first calculate the value of the numbers with exponents. Then multiply.

A. 16 * 5 * 3 = 240
B. 8 * 15 * 2 = 240
C. 27 * 5 * 2 = 270
D. 8 * 10 * 3 = 240

---

83 –   C. 18/37

There are 18 odd numbers between 0 and 36. The ball has an equal chance of landing in any of the 37 pockets. So the probability of the ball landing in an odd number is 18/37. (0 is technically considered an even number, but that is not relevant to this question.)

---

84 –   B. y^2

To divide numbers that have the same base and different exponents, keep the base the same and subtract the exponent of the divisor from the exponent of the dividend (in this case, 5 – 3). The answer is $y^{(5-3)}$, or y^2.

---

85 –   B. 70

Try each of the answers to see if it fits the requirements in the question. The numbers divisible by both 5 and 7 are 35, 70, 105, 140, 175…

The multiples of 6 are 6, 12, 18, 24, 30, 36, 42, 48, 54, 60, 66, 72, 78…

Since 70 – 66 = 4 the correct number is 70.

---

86 –   C. 2,3,4

The two shorter sides of a triangle must always add up to more than the longest side.

---

87 –   A. $33,500

Janet has a total of $105,000 in her accounts. 70% of that amount (her goal for her stock investments) is $73,500. To reach that goal, she would have to move $33,500 from bonds to stocks.

---

88 –   D. 432

Each machine can produce 12 parts per minute (96 ÷ 8). Multiply 12 by 12 (number of machines) by 3 (number of minutes).

---

89 –   B. 65

The average of 25, 35, and 120 is 60. 60 is 10 more than the average of the second set of numbers, so the average of the second set of numbers must be 50. The three numbers in the second set of numbers must add up to 150. Subtract 40 and 45 from 150 to get the answer, which is 65.

---

90 –   C. 5

Use x to represent the number of women on the board. Then the number of men is $x + 3$. So:

$$x + (x + 3) = 13$$
$$2x + 3 = 13$$

To isolate $2x$ on one side of the equation, subtract 3 from both sides.

$$2x = 10$$
$$x = 5$$

---

91 –   B. y = –2/3x + 2

The formula for a linear equation is y = *mx* + *b*, where *m* is the slope of the line to be graphed, and *b* is the y-intercept (the point where the line crosses the y axis).

The slope of the line in this graph is negative because it is moving downward from left to right. So the number before the x will be negative. Answers A and D cannot be correct answers.

The slope of the line is expressed as rise/run.

The slope of this line is –2/3 because it crosses the y-axis at 2 and the x-axis at 3. The y-intercept is 2. The correct equation must therefore be y = $-^2/_3$x + 2.

---

92 –   A. 9

Begin by subtracting –3 from both sides of the equation. (This is the same as adding +3). So:

$$\frac{4}{9}X = 4$$

Now, to isolate x on one side of the equation, divide both sides by 4/9. (To divide by a fraction, invert the fraction and multiply.

$$\frac{9}{4} * \frac{4}{9} X = \frac{4}{1} * \frac{9}{4}$$

You are left with $X = \dfrac{36}{4} = 9$.

---

93 –   B. x = 21, y = 2

The simplest way to solve this system of equations is to begin by eliminating one of the variables. Since the *x* variables have the same coefficient, they will be easier to eliminate. Subtract all the lined-up terms in one equation from all the lined-up terms in the other.

$$x - 3y = 15$$
$$- \underline{(x + 2y = 25)}$$
$$- 5y = -10$$

Now you can solve for *y*.

$$-5y = -10$$
$$y = 2$$

Replace *y* in the original equation with 2.

$$x - 3(2) = 15$$
$$x - 6 = 15$$
$$x = 21$$

Check your answer by substituting your determined values of x and y into both original equations.

---

94 – D. 1

If the y intercept of the depicted line is reduced by 1, the line would cross the y axis at 2. The slope of a line is defined as rise over run. You might also describe the slope of a line as the change in y over the change in x. If the y intercept is changed to 2, the slope of the line would then be 2/2, which is equal to 1. The slope of this line is positive because it is moving upward from left to right.

---

95 – C. $x = 12, y = 2$

The first step in solving this system of equations is to eliminate one of the variables. If one of the variables had the same coefficient in both equations, you could do this by subtracting one equation from the other. But both the x and y have different coefficients in the two equations. Therefore, you will have to make the coefficients of one variable the same by multiplying one of the equations by a number. In this case, the simplest thing to do is to multiply the first equation by 2.

$$2 \, (x - 2y = 8) = 2x - 4y = 16$$

Now you can subtract all the lined up terms in one equation from all the lined up terms in the other.

$$2x - 4y = 16$$
$$- \, (2x + 6y = 36)$$
$$- 10y = -20$$

Now you can solve for y.

$$-10y = -20$$
$$y = 2$$

Replace y in the original equation with 2.

$$x - 2(2) = 8$$
$$x - 4 = 8$$
$$x = 12$$

Check your answer by substituting your determined values of x and y into both original equations.

---

96 – B. $x = -1/2$ or -4

This is called a quadratic equation. All quadratic equations have this form:

$$ax^2 + bx + c = 0$$

In a quadratic equation, x is a variable; and a, b, and c are known values.

To solve this type of equation, you need to use the quadratic formula:

$$X = \frac{-b \pm \sqrt{b^2 - 4ac}}{2a}$$

Replace a, b, and c in this equation with the values in the equation you are solving:

$$X = \frac{-9 \pm \sqrt{9^2 - 4(2)(4)}}{2(2)}$$

Simplify the equation:

$$X = \frac{-9 \pm \sqrt{49}}{4}$$

$$X = \frac{-9 \pm 7}{4}$$

$$X = \frac{-2}{4} \text{ or } \frac{-16}{4}$$

$$X = -\frac{1}{2} \text{ or } -4$$

Quadratic equations may have two possible solutions.

---

97 –   **D.** $x = -\frac{1}{2} \text{ or } -2\frac{1}{2}$

This is called a quadratic equation. All quadratic equations have this form:

$$ax^2 + bx + c = 0$$

In a quadratic equation, x is a variable and a, b, and c are known values.

To solve this type of equation, you need to use the quadratic formula:

$$X = \frac{-b \pm \sqrt{b^2 - 4ac}}{2a}$$

Replace a, b, and c in this equation with the values in the equation you are solving:

$$X = \frac{-12 \pm \sqrt{12^2 - 4(4)(5)}}{2(4)}$$

Simplify this equation:

$$X = \frac{-12 \pm \sqrt{64}}{8}$$

$$X = \frac{-12 \pm 8}{8}$$

$$X = \frac{-4}{8} \text{ or } \frac{-20}{8}$$

$$X = -\frac{1}{2} \text{ or } -2\frac{1}{2}$$

Quadratic equations may have two possible solutions.

---

98 –   A. 100

The prime numbers less than 25 are 2, 3, 5, 7, 11, 13, 17, 19, and 23. The number 1 is not considered a prime number. The sum is 100

---

99 –   C. 7/3

An improper fraction is a fraction whose numerator is greater than its denominator. To convert a mixed number, such as $2\frac{1}{3}$, to an improper fraction, multiply the whole number (2) by the denominator (3), then add the result to the numerator: $2\frac{1}{3} = \frac{7}{3}$

---

100 –   B. $xy = x + y + 6$

The product of the two numbers is x times y, or xy. Therefore, xy equals the sum of the two numbers $(x + y)$ plus 6.

---

101 –   C. 7

The perimeter of the rectangle is 28 (8 + 8 + 6 + 6). If the perimeter of the square is also 28, then the length of each of its sides must be 7.

INTERMEDIATE PRACTICE TEST: SCIENCE

1- B. Cilia

Cilia that are located on the outer membrane of bronchial epithelial cells are motile hairlike extension whose motion tends to move substances out of the airways toward the pharynx. Microvilli are found on the villi of intestinal epithelial cells. Flagella are found on sperm cells, but no other cells in the human body. Dendrites are thin branching cellular extensions of neuron cell membranes.

2- D. bile; small intestine

Fats molecules are primarily hydrocarbon in content and are therefore not soluble in water. To absorb fats the liver produces bile that is secreted into the duodenum. Fats are soluble in bile so bile is able to break large fat globules into smaller droplets which can be more easily absorbed into the body. The process of fat globule dissolution is call emulsification. Amylase is a digestive enzyme that breaks down certain carbohydrates.

3- D. intercellular membrane binding

The role of T-helper cells in immune responses involves the binding of membrane bound molecules, usually receptors or membrane bound antigens or antibodies between the T-helper cells and other immune system cells including B-cells and antigen-presenting cells, such as macrophages. T-helper cells can produce antibodies that bind to their own membranes, but do not produce antibodies that are released into the circulation (B-cells do this). T-helper cells do not directly cause lysis of other dells and do not engage in phagocytosis.

4- A. It passes through capillaries before returning to the internal chambers of the heart

Rationale: Blood is pumped out of the heart through either the pulmonic valve as deoxygenated blood to the pulmonary artery or secondly, through the aortic valve as oxygenated blood to the aorta. All blood, once it leaves the heart, must pass through capillaries before it returns to the internal chambers of the heart

5- D. continuously throughout the entire respiratory cycle

Deoxygenated blood is pumped through alveolar capillaries continuously throughout the respiratory cycle. If oxygen were not diffusing into the capillaries throughout each of the stages of the inspiratory cycle, the blood passing through the alveolar capillaries would not be oxygenated. This deoxygenated blood would return to the heart and mix with oxygenated blood, lowering the oxygen saturation level of the blood that is then pumped out of the heart through the aorta. Blood exiting the heart through the aorta is nearly 100% saturated so there is no inspiratory phase where oxygen is not passing into the circulatory system through the alveoli into their surrounding capillaries.

6- A. sensory input

The integrative functions of the nervous system occur in the brain, where sensory input is utilized to create memories and to help generate thought processes. This does not require hormonal regulation. Effector cells are cells that carry out instructions from the nervous system at locations throughout the body. This is not classified as integrative neurological function. Spinal cord reflexes are, for the most part, independent of the central nervous system and are not required for integrative functions.

7- B. CCK and secretin

Pepsinogen is a proenzyme released by the stomach and trypsinogen is a proenzyme released by the pancreas. CCK (cholecystokinin) is a hormone that stimulates the release of bile from the gall bladder and secretin is hormone that stimulates the release of bicarbonate from the pancreas. Both CCK and secretin are released by the duodenum.

8- C. production of antibodies

The innate immune system generates non-specific immune responses. Phagocytosis of foreign cells by macrophages, the stimulation of fever by the release of interleukins, and the release of and response to cytokines by cells involved in the innate immune responses is triggered by a wide variety of infectious agents or chemicals generated by tissue injury. the innate immune responses are then carried out through biochemical pathways and cell activities that do not require the participation of antibodies or the recognition of a specific antigens. Antibodies are produced by B-cells, which are required for activity of the humoral category of the body's adaptive immune system. B-cells do not participate in the innate immune responses.

9- A. The heart if ventral to the esophagus

The term ventral means toward the umbilical (belly button) abdominal wall versus the opposite direction, dorsal, which means, in this positional terminology, toward the spine. Proximal means toward the midline of the body, so it also can be interpreted as toward or closer to the spine, but this is contrasted with the opposite of proximal, which is described by the term distal, meaning away from the spine. Medial is used to describe relative locations toward any central axis of the body with the opposite relationship described by the term lateral, meaning to the side of that which is medial. Rostral indicates a relative position closer to the skull with the term caudal meaning a relative position that is closer to the base of the spine.

10- A. the liver

Urea is water-soluble, non-toxic molecule synthesized for the purpose of ridding the body of waste products generated by the catabolism of nitrogen containing compounds such as nucleic acids and proteins. Although urea is excreted through the kidneys it is synthesized by liver parenchymal cells.

11- D. the large intestine

All organs of the body must receive a direct arterial supply of oxygenated blood. The lungs also receive deoxygenated blood through the pulmonary artery, which is then oxygenated as it passes through alveolar capillaries. The heart receives deoxygenated blood through the superior and inferior vena cava veins which empty into the right atrium. The liver receives deoxygenated blood through the hepatic portal vein, which carries blood that has passed through capillaries in the small intestines. The large intestine, along with most of the other organs or organ regions of the body, receives supplies of oxygenated blood only.

12- B. the diaphragm

One is not expected to know the names of all of the voluntary muscles in the body, but the major voluntary muscles, such as the biceps are expected knowledge. the masseters are the muscles that cause the lower jaw to close. This is beyond expected knowledge but it is a higher level of anatomical knowledge that is not specifically, but as a category of superior mastery, included to distinguish the top levels of performance. At the expected knowledge level is that the diaphragm is the muscle that generates inhalation, that one can for brief periods of time voluntarily inhale or suppress inhalation but usually the inhalation process is involuntary, and always involuntary when one is asleep.

13- C. the small intestines

This question is often missed because most students know that the primary role of the large intestine is to absorb water. Nevertheless, 80% of water that passes through the digestive system is absorbed through the small intestine.

14- B. natural killer (NK) cells

Perforins are small molecules that are secreted by natural killer cells. They insert themselves into the cell membrane of the natural killer's target cell - the cell that the natural killer wants to kill - and arrange themselves to form a hole or perforation in the target cell's cell membrane. When sufficient quantities of these hole have been created. the target cell's internal contents leak away, its internal environment is increasingly diluted and its internal organelles are destabilized then rendered inoperable, and finally the target cell dies.

15- C. inadequate intake during childhood development can lead to the disease kwashiorkor

Kwashiorkor is a severe form of malnourishment which is usually fatal. It is specifically the result of inadequate protein intake that occurs children usually after the age of 18 months. Vegetarians can obtain all required dietary protein through non-animal or animal product sources -rice and legumes are sufficient for example. There are nine essential amino acids which must be obtained through the diet. The remaining amino acids can be synthesized by the body. The breakdown of proteins begins within the stomach.

16- A. Eubacteria and Archaebacteria

Before the introduction of the broadest category of living organisms, domains, kingdoms were the broadest category. Subsequently extensive genetic and biochemical analysis of species that had been classified as bacteria were found to differ from other bacteria in more fundamental ways that other bacteria differ from organisms in other kingdoms. This lead to the creation of the higher level category of "domain", with the Bacteria kingdom divided into two separate domains The Eubacteria and the Archaea or Archaebacteria. All other organisms are now assigned to the third domain, Eukarya.

17- B. Mutations in the germ line cells of the fertile members of the species must be able to occur

Without the possibility of the occurrence of mutations in DNA that can be passed to offspring, which is germline DNA found only in germline cells, no new genes or variations of genes in the form of alleles could be created. All offspring would have genes contained only in the genepool of the previous generation. One might argue that speciation could occur for a limited amount of time and to a limited extent by adaptation through natural selection for fitter combination of alleles that were already present in the previous generation's gene pool. This is actually an invalid argument however because it overlooks the fact that without germline mutations, there is no mechanism for the production of any alleles of genes to begin with.

18- C. a phosphate group, a pentose sugar and a nitrogenous base

In both RNA and DNA molecules, the backbone of a continuous single DNA or RNA molecular chain is an alternating sequence of cyclic 5-carbon sugars (pentoses) bonded to phosphate groups ($PO4$). each pentose sugar is also bonded to one of five possible nitrogenous bases. nitrogenous bases in nucleic acids are small, cyclic nitrogen-containing molecules consisting of either one or two rings. A nucleotide is defined as a molecular subunit consisting of one of these nitrogenous base that bonded to a nucleic acid pentose sugar and a phosphate group that is also bonded to the same pentose sugar. Any DNA or RNA segment can be built entirely from combinations of theses nucleotide subunits.

19- D. Some, but not all, eukaryotic cells have chloroplasts, but no prokaryotic cells have chloroplasts

Prokaryotic cells do not possess a nucleus. Prokaryotic cell DNA is organized into a structures called a nucleoid which analogous to a nucleus in eukaryotic cells. Cell walls are present in eukaryotic kingdoms of Plantae and Fungi and some organisms of the kingdom Protozoa, but not in any organisms in the kingdom Animalia. All organisms of the kingdom Plantae and some of the kingdom Protozoa have chloroplasts. No prokaryotes have chloroplasts. Every living cell contains ribosomes.

20- B. ribosomes

Ribosomes are protein complexes that may be free-floating within a cell's cytoplasm or, at times, attached to a cell's endoplasmic reticulum. It is simply a fact that they do not possess outer membranes, or, in fact, any membranes whatsoever. There is strong evidence that mitochondria, chloroplasts and the nuclei of eukaryotic cells evolved from prokaryotic cells that were ingested by other prokaryotic cells but survived and evolved to their present state within the evolutionary descendants of these cells. This is a compelling explanation for why these organelles possess encapsulating membranes.

21- D. The mRNA segment base sequence is identical to the complementary DNA strand segment of the gene base sequence except that uracil is substituted for thymine in the mRNA base sequence

An important and common misconception regarding RNA transcriptions of a gene is that the RNA transcription is a copy of the DNA gene segment except that uracil is substituted for thymine in the RNA sequence. In fact, the RNA segment is the compliment of the gene sequence, except that in the RNA transcript, uracil is substituted for by thymine.

22- A. Individual tissue layers begin to form

By definition, the gastrulation stage of development is the stage where individual tissue layers begin to form. The first multipotent stem cells begin to appear, and the four fundamental cell types begin to differentiate before the gastrulation stage. The organ differentiation stage occurs after the gastrulation stage

23- A. prophase, G1 and G2

The normal somatic cell cycle is divided into the mitotic and the non-mitotic stages. The non-mitotic stage is referred to as interphase. Interphase is divided into three subphases, G1, S, and G2. The mitotic stage of the cell cycle is divided into four stages; prophase, metaphase, anaphase and telophase. Cytokinesis refers to the physical separation of a cell into two daughter cells. This occurs during anaphase and telophase of mitosis in a normal somatic cell cycle and during anaphase and telophase of meiosis I and II of gamete cell production in the germ-line cell cycle.

24- B. individual tetrads align

Tetrads are formations of closely aligned homologous chromosome pairs where each chromosome is in the form where it consists of two identical sister chromatids. Tetrads only form during meiosis I. they can exchange chromatid segments as they are pulled apart during anaphase of meiosis I This is referred to as crossing over. When crossing over occurs, 2 new hybrid chromosomes are formed.

25- B. 6

During photosynthesis the following chemical reaction occurs:

$6CO_2 + 6H_2O$ + sunlight --> $C_6H_{12}O_6 + 6O_2$. You should be able to balance simple chemical reactions and to know that photosynthesis uses carbon dioxide and water to produce glucose and oxygen. This gives an initial unbalanced reaction of _CO + _H_2O --> $C_6H_{12}O_6$ + _O_2. There are 12 hydrogens in glucose so there must be $6H_2O$ molecules on the left side of the reaction. there are 6 carbon atoms in glucose so there must be 6 CO_2 molecules on the left side of the equation. The total number of Oxygen atoms required is 6 from 6 H_2O and 6x2=12 from $6CO_2$. This gives a total of 6+12=18 Oxygen atoms. Six oxygen atoms are used to form one glucose molecule leaving 12 or 12/2=6 O_2 molecules on the right side of the balanced equation.

26- B. A single, unique three-base codon will code for only one single, unique type of amino acid

This is a question that is commonly answered incorrectly. DNA is comprised, in part, of a linear sequence of nitrogenous base subunits. these subunits can be any of four different nitrogenous bases. These bases transmit genetic information in the form of 3-base unit sequences that are called codons. Statistically there are 64 possible 3-base sequences that can be constructed from a combination of these four different DNA bases.

27- B. identical genotypes only

Perfectly identical twins will have exactly the same genotypes. They may have different phenotypes because phenotypic expression is often dependent on the environment. Identical twins raised in different environments likely have obvious phenotypic differences.

28- B. H_2CO_3 is a weak acid

A strong base in that results from the deprotonation of an acid will strongly accept hydrogen ion, so the reverse reaction is favored, meaning the acid is preferentially more protonated than deprotonated at equilibrium This is the definition of a weak acid.

29- C. electromagnetic energy

Although the sun does emit vast amounts of electrons and protons in the form of the solar wind, the energy carried by the solar wind that reaches the earth is miniscule in comparison to the energy that is emitted by the sun in the form of electromagnetic waves that is received by the earth. The majority of this electromagnetic radiation is in the visible light wavelength spectrum.

30- A. a 5 kg mass, at rest, 10 m above the surface of the earth

Gravitational potential energy of an object is given by the equation $Fg=mgh$, where m is the object's mass and h is the object's height above the surface of the earth. The velocity of an object contributes nothing to the object's gravitational potential energy. For choice C, the object is actually below the surface of the earth so in a sense it actually has negative potential energy. For choice D, the object is at the surface of the earth so its potential energy is zero regardless of its mass. Between choices A and B, the mass of the objects is irrelevant because they are equal. The object in A has twice the potential energy compared to the object in B because object A's height above the earth's surface is twice that of object B's height.

31- B. connective tissue

An organized functional collection of a single type of cell is considered to be a tissue. Adipose cells (fat cells) are classified as a type of connective cell and therefore adipose cell tissue is connective tissue. A syncytium is a collection of cells that have to some extent fused such that cytoplasm can circulate throughout the entire collection of cells, A gland is an organized cell structure that secretes substance through a duct.

32- C. increases the rate of the reaction; increasing the activation energy

The efficiency of a reaction is the actual yield compared to the theoretical yield of products of the reaction. This is a function of the conditions under which the reaction occurs, but it is not affected by the presence of a catalyst. A catalyst increases the rate of a reaction by lowering the activation energy of the reaction. The activation energy is the difference between the energy of the reactants and the highest energy transition state between reactants and products. Lowering the energy of this transition state increases the probability that reactants will have sufficient energy to achieve the transition state so that the reaction can proceed to the final product state.

33- A. 1s2 2s2 2p6

The electron subshells of an atom beginning with the lowest energy subshells are the 1s, 2s, 2p, 3s, 3d and 3p subshells. The s subshells are filled when they contain 2 electrons. The p subshells are filled when they contain a total of 6 electrons. Neon, with an atomic number of 10 will in have neutral atoms with ten electrons and in the lowest energy state these will fill the lowest available energy levels. This corresponds to an electron configuration of 1s2 2s2 2p6

34- C. The enzyme has increased its effect on the rate of a chemical reaction

Enzyme activity is quantified, for the biochemical reaction that the enzyme catalyzes, as the amount of product generated per unit time. In general, it indicates how fast a reaction is occurring. The major factors that affect an enzyme's ability to increase the rate of a reaction are temperature, pH at which the reaction occurs and concentrations of the reactants and products of the reaction.

35- B. ammonia, blood, orange juice

Sulphuric acid is a strong acid so it will have a very low pH relative to either orange juice or vinegar which are weak acids. All acids by definition will have a pH that is lower than water. Water is neutral by definition, with a pH of 7.0. Blood is nearly neutral but slightly basic with a pH of 7.4 which is higher than any acid pH. Ammonia is a strong base so its pH will higher than any acid pH or any substances with a pH that is close to neutral pH.

36- A. The alkane contains 4 less hydrogen atoms than does the alkyne

Rationale: When an alkane is converted to an alkyne, two adjacent carbons in the alkane each break the bonds with two of their bonded hydrogens and then form two new carbon-carbon bonds between the two adjacent carbons resulting in the formation of a carbon-carbon triple bond. In the process the alkane loses the four hydrogens whose carbon-hydrogen bonds were broken during the triple bond formation process.

37- B. the adrenal gland

Steroid hormones are produced in the adrenal gland, in the gonads primarily. The pancreas produces insulin and glucagon which are peptide hormones. The thyroid hormones are also peptide hormones. The thymus is the site of T-cell maturation. It does not secrete any hormones.

38- B. 2O2 + 8e- ---> 4O-2

In oxidation-reduction reactions the reactants give product molecules that have covalent bonds, but there is a large difference in the electronegativities between the bonded atoms in the product molecules. The atoms in these molecules are not ions but they can be thought of as having strong ionic character, and that they undergo electron loss or electron acquisition as shown for the two molecules of oxygen in the answer choice B. Within a common solution environment these ions are never actually present, but if the reactants are separated into different reaction vessels and connected by an electrically conductive wire and a salt bridge, electrons will flow from the less electronegative species to the more electronegative species through the wire. This is how chemical batteries are constructed

39- B. The temperature of the liquid bromine will remain constant

The question describes a liquid that is undergoing a phase transition from liquid to gas. During phase transitions that require the input of energy (heat), the energy applied to the particles undergoing the transition does not result in any increase in temperature. Instead, the applied energy is consumed by the processes that allow particles to transition between the two phases.

40- A. the same type of

There are no different types of intermolecular bonding that occur among water molecules in the solid phase compared to the liquid phase. The difference is that the kinetic energy of water molecules in the solid phase is insufficient to overcome the intermolecular bonds that hold the water molecules in a fixed position relative to surrounding water molecules. In the liquid phase, water molecules have sufficient kinetic energy to change position within the liquid but insufficient energy to completely break free of intermolecular bonds and thus become gas phase water molecules.

41- C. class; order

The hierarchy of modern taxonomic classification categories, beginning with the broadest, most inclusive category is: domain, kingdom, phylum, class, order, family, genus and species.

42- C. every functional gene can be transcribed into a mRNA molecule

A single chromosome can exist in two different forms. In the singular form it contains a full set of genes, there may be more than one copy of a given gene and there may be more than one version of a given gene - which is called an allele located on the chromosome. It is not true that there are always two copies or two alleles of a gene on this version of a chromosome. In preparation for cell division, a copy of the single chromosome is made resulting in a version of the chromosome that consists of two identical sister chromatids. In this version there are always at least two copies of every gene, but not at least two alleles for every gene. Only one strand of a double -stranded DNA molecule contains genes. The other strand contains the complementary sequence of the DNA's genes, but this strand cannot be transcribed into RNA that will code for any gene proteins. By definition, a gene is a sequence of DNA bases that can be translated into a protein and this requires that every gene be capable of being first transcribed into a messenger RNA molecule.

43- B. UCG AUG GGC

In DNA, complementary base pairing occurs between adenine (A) and thymine (T) and between guanine (G) and cytosine (C). In RNA, the same complementary base relationship is true except that the complementary base of adenine is uracil (U) rather than thymine. The base sequence in choice B correctly identifies the complementary base sequence for RNA to the base sequence for DNA that is given within the question.

44- D. nucleoli

Nucleoli are located with the nucleus of cells. These are the organelles that are responsible for the construction of ribosomes. Peroxisomes and lysosomes are intracellular vesicles that contain specific types of substances, but they are not involved in ribosome construction. Ribosomes are attached to the endoplasmic reticular membranes in rough endoplasmic reticulum, but they are not constructed by the endoplasmic reticulum.

45- C. RNA polymerase

Ribosomes are the structures that physically assemble proteins by reading RNA base sequences and connecting amino acids to form a chain of amino acids, which is, by definition, a protein. RNA polymerase is the structure, in the form of an enzyme complex, that physically assembles messenger RNA molecules by reading DNA base sequences and connecting nucleotides to form a chain of nucleotides, which becomes the messenger RNA molecule.

46- D. Replication of both strands occurs simultaneously

The process of replication of double-stranded DNA begins with the breaking of hydrogen bonds between a small sequence of complementary base pairs at a single site on the DNA molecule This creates a gap within the DNA that allows a DNA polymerase enzyme complex to enter and to begin adding nucleotides with complementary bases to both the sense and antisense strands of the original DNA, The process differs somewhat between the two strands, but replication proceeds simultaneously on both strands.

47- B. centrosomes and chromosomes

The role of spindle fibers during mitosis is to separate the sister chromatids of each chromosome and then draw one of each chromatid pair to opposite sides of the dividing cell. This occurs by the connection of microtubules to the central region of the chromosome and then to either of the two centrosomes located on opposite sides of the cell. The microtubules then begin to shorten and move, along with an attached sister chromatid, towards either one or the other centrosomes. The process of cytokinesis follows and results in the production of two daughter cells, each containing one set of the sister chromatids.

48- B. absorption of sunlight

Chlorophyll molecules are located in the chloroplasts of cells that are capable of photosynthesis. Chlorophyll molecules absorb visible light wavelength photons and convert the photon energy into chemical energy stored in the bonds of carbohydrate molecules

49- A. purines and pyrimidines

Purines and pyrimidines are the two structural categories of nitrogenous bases that are found in DNA and RNA. The purines are guanine and adenine; the pyrimidines are thymine cytosine and uracil. The major structural difference between the two is that purines have a two-ring structure and pyrimidines have a one-ring structure.

50- A. 1 base error per 1000 genes

Without error correction mechanisms, this baseline level of error in DNA replication would result in extinction of a species within a few or possibly only one generation. Choice D is the final estimated error rate in human DNA after replication and subsequent error corrections of DNA by various repair mechanisms.

51- D. incomplete dominance

An example of a genetic disease with incomplete dominance is sickle cell disease. The severe form of the disease, sickle cell anemia, is the homozygous form the disease. Sickle cell trait is the heterozygous and milder form of the disease. In some types of abnormal hemoglobin genetic diseases there are not one but four genes that can have disease mutations and there are specific hemoglobin genetic diseases that can have four disease variants with severity ranging from normal to fatal.

52- D. 5.0 m/s

Kinetic energy for an object with mass m and velocity v is given by the equation $KE = \frac{1}{2}(mv^2)$. To solve for the velocity of the object, rearrange the equation to $v = (2KE//m)^{\frac{1}{2}}$. This gives $v = (250/10)^{\frac{1}{2}}$ which reduces to the square root of 25 which is equal to 5, The units of velocity are m/s, therefore the velocity of the object is 5 m/s

53- A. the electron charge magnitude to the proton charge magnitude

So far no experiment has ever detected any difference between the magnitude of the charge of a proton and an electron. Atomic theory also predicts that the charge magnitudes are exactly equal. Therefore, the ratio of the magnitudes of the electron and proton charge is exactly one. The masses of protons and neutrons are very similar but not equal, the neutron is slightly more massive than the proton so the proton to neutron mass ratio will be slightly less than one. The electron mass is thousands of times less than the proton mass so the electron to proton mass ratio will be nowhere close to one.

54- B. No element's atomic number is larger than the element's atomic mass

The atomic number of an element is equal to the number of protons in the individual nuclei of atoms of the element. This is always a whole number value. Every element includes atoms whose nuclei possess both protons and neutrons, including hydrogen, which has two isotopes, deuterium and tritium which have one and two nuclear neutrons respectively. The atomic mass of an element is equal to the average number of protons and neutrons in the nuclei of atoms of the element. Therefore, the atomic number of an element can never exceed the atomic mass of the element.

55- B. epithelial

Epithelial tissues are the tissues that are exposed to the outside environment and to the contents of the digestive tract. They are therefore exposed to the greatest mechanical and chemical stresses of the major tissue types. Without a high regenerative capacity, epithelial cells would not be able to serve their protective functions in the skin and absorption functions in the intestines. In humans who have reached adulthood, connective, nervous and blood tissues have comparatively low or even no regenerative capacity.

56- A. the left atrium

The right and left ventricles are thick-walled muscular structures that are capable of generating much higher blood pressure during contraction than the comparatively thin-wall right and left atria. During ventricular contraction, the atrioventricular valves (the tricuspid and mitral valves) seal the passages between the atria and ventricles so that the atria are not exposed to the high blood pressures generated in the ventricles. The pulmonary artery is the outflow route for the right ventricle and therefore experiences peak blood pressures that are nearly as high as the right ventricle peak blood pressure.

57- C. alveolar airspaces

The respiratory airways are all continuous with each other, forming a respiratory tree beginning with the pharynx which is open to outside air at the mouth and nose. The outside air has by far the lowest concentration of carbon dioxide compared to any respiratory airspaces. The highest concentration of carbon dioxide in the respiratory airways occurs in the alveoli, where carbon dioxide is diffusing out of the bloodstream. The carbon dioxide concentrations in all other regions of the respiratory airways will vary depending on whether inhalation or exhalation are occurring, but gases always diffuse from regions of higher concentration to regions of lower concentration, so it is not possible for any region of the airways to experience a peak carbon dioxide concentration level that is higher than the region where carbon dioxide first diffuses into the airway, namely the alveolar airspaces.

58- C. parasympathetic; increased peristalsis

The sympathetic division of the autonomic nervous system generates "fight or flight" category of physiological responses including the redirection of blood flow to skeletal muscles resulting in increased blood flow to skeletal muscles. The parasympathetic division of the autonomic nervous system generates the "rest and digest" physiological responses including the increase of peristaltic activity in the intestines. The central nervous system can trigger either the sympathetic or parasympathetic responses depending on the brain's perception of the nature of the external environment.

59- D. Secretin

Secretin is a hormone produced by the duodenum that stimulate the pancreas to release bicarbonate ion into the lumen of the duodenum. This occurs before the contents of the stomach are released into the duodenum. The stomach contents have a pH close to that of battery acid. The bicarbonate ion secreted by the pancreas is a base that neutralizes the stomach acids. Without secretin there would be no release of bicarbonate ion into the duodenum. When the contents of the stomach then entered the duodenum they would not be neutralized by bicarbonate. The result would be severe chemical injury to the duodenum caused by the stomach contents due to their high acidity.

60- B. diapedesis

Diapedesis is the process where mobile cells such as certain types of white blood cells are able to squeeze between lymph vessel and blood vessel wall cells and then exit into the surrounding tissue. Diaphoresis is a medical term for sweating. Chemotaxis is the movement of a cell or organism along an increasing liquid-phase chemical gradient. Facilitated diffusion is the term for chemical movements down a concentration gradient that is aided by the presence of cell membrane channels and other cellular constructions.

61- C. the brain and the spinal cord

The body at the most general level can be divided into the dorsal and ventral cavities. The dorsal cavity includes the cranial cavity and the spinal canal. The ventral cavity is divided by the diaphragm into the thoracic and abdominal cavities. The pharynx and larynx are not in any true anatomical cavity of the body. They are regions of the airway which is technically an out branching of a tube that runs through the body. The kidneys are covered by tissues and are not considered to be in the abdominal cavity but rather buried in the dorsolateral walls of the abdominal cavity. The heart and lungs are in the thoracic cavity.

62- A. vasoconstriction and vasodilation

Although the blood is usually at a higher temperature than the air outside of the body, dilation of vessels in the skin increases blood flow to the skin. Heat can flow from the blood to the atmosphere in the form of latent heat absorbed by sweat on the skin surface which is then carried off by water contained in sweat as it evaporates from the surface of the skin. In high humidity conditions, sweat evaporation will decrease or, as humidity levels approach 100%, cease entirely. Under these circumstances the body will be unable to rid itself of excess heat by this mechanism. Heat loss, conversely can be minimized by vasoconstriction of vessels within the skin; this minimizes the transfer heat from the bloodstream and out of the body to the outside environment

63- B. The thoracic cavity increases its volume

The diaphragm separates the thoracic cavity from the abdominal cavity. It is dome shaped and has a convex surface within the thoracic cavity. Contraction of the diaphragm causes the diaphragm to flatten, which expands the volume of the thoracic cavity. This lowers intrathoracic pressure resulting in a pressure gradient compared to atmospheric pressure. This results in the flow of air from outside of the body into the airways and lungs.

64- D. a ganglion

A synapse is a junction between two neurons where neurotransmitters from one neuron are passed to the other neuron. In the macroscopic central nervous system some collections of neurons are referred to as nuclei such as the solitary nucleus and the nucleus accumbens, but no such term is used for collections of neurons outside of the central nervous system. Nerve tracts are composed primarily of the axons of neurons, not neuron cell bodies. All organized collections of neurons outside of the nervous system are referred to as ganglia.

65- A. intrinsic factor

Intrinsic factor is produced by parietal cell located in the stomach and is required for the absorption of vitamin B12 by the small intestine. In humans, autoimmune disease and other conditions can inhibit the production or activity of intrinsic factor, resulting in vitamin B12 deficiency. The production of red blood cells requires vitamin B12. The major consequence of such deficiency is anemia, an insufficiency of red blood cells. In severe cases this form of anemia can be fatal if untreated by vitamin

B12 injections.

66- D. consumption of breast milk

Passive immunity is a short-term type of immunity that is acquired by the acquisition of pre-formed antibodies either through natural means as antibodies contained in breast milk, or artificially in the form of medically produced antitoxins or preformed antibodies to other disease causing agents. disease causing agents. Vaccines generate an immune response where the antibodies are produced by one's own body, this is a form of active immunity. The process described in choice C is a possible method to suppress an immune response to Rh antigens located on red blood cells.

67- C. argon (Ag)

An atom with fifteen electrons and a net charge of -3 will have three additional electrons in its neutral state for a total of 18 atoms. This corresponds to a nucleus with 18 protons. Atoms with 18 protons are by definition atoms of the element atomic number 18, which is the element argon.

68- C. is present in an equal number of catalytic units before the beginning of and after the completion of the catalytic reaction

By definition a catalyst remains unchanged by the reaction that it catalyzes. During the reaction it may undergo a chemical change, but this is reversed before or very soon after the completion of each round of the reaction.

69- D. Every electron added to the n=2 level electron shell experiences exactly the same effective nuclear charge

Electrons at the n=1 level are exposed to the full positive nuclear charge of their parent atom. Electrons at progressively higher n levels experience a progressively weaker nuclear charge because they are farther away from the nucleus and because intervening filled lower n level electron shells partially shield or block the outer electrons from the experiencing the full nuclear charge. This shielding does not occur among electrons in the same n electron shell level, therefore every electron at a given n level experiences the same nuclear charge, regardless of how many electrons occupy the n level.

70- A. sodium (Na)

Potassium is a group I element on the periodic table. Group I elements have one valence electron which is very easily ionized by other more electronegative atoms. After this first ionization however all other electrons in are in filled n=1, 2, 3 and 4 shells. These electrons are held extremely tightly. The only second ionization energy that would be comparable to the second ionization energy of potassium would be a second ionization that also resulted in extracting an electron from a completely filled n electron shell level. Calcium and magnesium each have 2 valence electrons so their second ionization do not require extraction of an electron from a filled n level. Sodium and rubidium are also group I elements so a second ionization does require the extraction of an electron from a filled n level The strongest held of all of these electrons would be sodium, because the extraction would be from the n=3 level, for potassium the extraction would occur at the n=4 level For rubidium the extraction would occur at the =5 levels. The lower the n level the more strongly electrons are attracted to the atomic nucleus, therefore the ionization energy is higher for electrons in lower n levels compared to higher n levels

___

71- B. Intercellular transfer of DNA

Pili are hollow tubes through which bacteria connect and exchange DNA. The other choices describe functions that require microtubules, another type of structural building unit that is not biochemically similar to pili.

___

72- C. 4.0 C

Water is almost unique among molecular compounds in that its maximum density at atmospheric pressure occurs in the liquid rather than the solid phase and the liquid phase in general is denser than the solid phase. This is fortunate, since if the reverse were true, ice would sink to the bottom of bodies of water, eventually this would lead to the freezing of nearly all bodies of water on earth including lakes seas and even oceans. For the choices above A and B are negative values for degrees Celsius and by definition represent water in the solid phase at atmospheric pressure. For choice D water at atmospheric pressure is a gas, since the boiling point of water is defined as a temperature equal to 100 degrees Celsius. The gas phase of water is of course much less dense than the liquid or solid phases of water.

___

73- C. the enzyme's activity for the reverse reaction will progressively increase to a maximum level as the concentrations of C and D increase

The activity of biological enzymes (the amount of products produced per unit time) are dependent on several factors, the most important of which are the concentration of the reactant and products of the reaction being catalyzed and the temperature and pH at which the reaction is occurring. If the enzyme can catalyze the reverse reacting the enzyme activity for the reverse reaction will increase as the concentrations of the products of the forward reaction (which are the reactants for the reverse reaction) increases. All enzymes have a maximum activity level, so further increase in the concentrations of C and D in the reaction will have no further effect on enzyme activity once the maximum activity is reached.

___

74- A. A neutral magnesium atom's atomic diameter is greater than and electronegativity is less than the atomic diameter and electronegativity of a neutral sulfur atom

Many properties of elements follow various trends in the periodic table. Among these are the atomic radius of elements and the electronegativity of elements. Magnesium and sulfur are in the same row in the periodic table, with magnesium located four columns to the left of sulfur. Among elements located in the same row in the periodic table, atomic diameter decreases from left to right and electronegativity increase from left to right. The exception to this is that the last element in the row on the right is a noble gas, which has the lowest electronegativity of all other elements in that row.

___

75- C. bone

The body requires large amounts of phosphorus which are used to create nucleic acids and ATP among many other functions. The largest reserves of phosphorus (and calcium) are stored in the mineral matrices of bones.

___

76- C. the lungs and the kidneys

The pH of blood is tightly controlled around an ideal level of 7.4. Metabolic processes produce organic acid that will lower blood pH and carbon dioxide in the blood will react with water to produce carbonic acid (H_2CO_3), a weak acid, which will also tend to decrease blood pH. The kidneys are the primary regulator of blood pH by several biochemical and physiologic methods. Removal of carbon dioxide from the blood by the lungs is also critical to maintaining optimum blood pH.

77- A. proofreading and mismatch repair only

The two error repair mechanisms that occur during replication of DNA are first proofreading repairs by DNA polymerase while it synthesizes new complementary DNA to the DNA that is being read by the DNA polymerase. Before DNA chains are completely replicated a second error correction mechanism called mismatch repair occurs through the actions of other repair proteins. This mechanism attempts to repair and replication errors not corrected by proofreading mechanisms. Excision repair occurs in DNA strands that are not undergoing replication. This mechanism does not operate while a cell is in mitosis or meiosis cell phases.

78- C. the pH of the solution multiplied by negative 1

The pH of a solution is defined as the negative log of the hydrogen ion concentration of the solution. Therefore, the reverse is true, the log of the hydrogen ion concentration of a solution must be the negative value of the pH of the solution, which is the pH of the solution multiplied by negative one.

79- B. C_nH_{2n}

All hydrocarbons that contain only single bonds are classified as alkanes. The general formula for alkanes is C_nH_{2n+2}. Alkenes are also hydrocarbons that have only single bonds with the exception that they also contain one carbon-carbon double bond per molecule. To form this second carbon-carbon bond resulting in a carbon-carbon double bond. Two adjacent carbons must each break a carbon-hydrogen bond to form the new carbon-carbon bond. The alkene will therefore have 2 less hydrogens than the corresponding alkane. For this reason, the general formula for an alkene is C_nH_{2n}.

80- A. CH_4

Rationale: Covalent bonds between atoms involve the sharing of electrons. In some molecules, such as elemental molecules such as H_2 and O_2 electron sharing between the two atoms is exactly equal. Usually in a covalent bond between different atoms, one atom has a higher electronegativity than the other and will draw electron density toward itself and away from the less electronegative atom. This unequal sharing results is a partial positive character to one end of the bond and a partial negative character to the other end of the bond. The covalent bond is now defined as having polarity. The greater the difference in electronegativity between the two covalently bonded atoms, the greater the polarity of the covalent bond. Of the choices above, the greatest difference in electronegativity between covalently bonded atoms occurs in the molecule HCl, since hydrogen is a participant in every covalent bond and chlorine is the most electronegative of all of the atoms present in the answer choices.

81- A. Prokaryote

Although the distinction between prokaryotes and eukaryotes is a fundamental distinction, prokaryote is not a taxonomic distinction. This is because, at the broadest taxonomic level, the domain level, there are three domains; Archaea (or Archaebacteria), Bacteria (or Eubacteria) and Eukarya. The definition of a prokaryote is an organism that lacks any cellular nuclei. This is the case for all organisms in both the Bacteria and Archaea domains. Therefor the prokaryote definition cannot be used as a more specific taxonomic subcategory since it is a universal characteristic of all organisms in more than one domain. Aves is the class of animals that includes all birds. Canis is the genus name that includes dogs and wolves. Ursidae is the animal family that includes bears.

82- A. phase transitions

Latent heat is a term for the energy required for substances to undergo a phase transition. The actual value of latent heat depends on the pressure under which the phase transition occurs. Examples of latent heat values include the heat of vaporization, referring to the heat required for a given mass of a substance to undergo a phase transition to the gas phase.

83- D. donate valence electrons to a collective valence electron level

In pure samples of transition metal elements, valence electrons, usually in the d and/or f subshells, are "delocalized" meaning they are free to move about among the metal atoms. These delocalized electrons form a collective valence electron level referred to as the conduction band. It is this delocalization phenomena that results in the high electrical conductivity of transition metal elements,

84- C. KCl; H_2O

The TEAS test expects one to recognize the most common strong acids and strong bases. In particular HCL is hydrochloric acid - a strong acid and KOH is potassium hydroxide - a strong base. HCl completely dissociates in water to form Cl^- and H^+ (the subscript "aq" indicates the reactants are reacting in an aqueous solution. An aqueous solution means that liquid water is the solvent) and KOH completely dissociates in water to form from K^+ and OH^-. H^+ and OH^- then combine to form H_2O and K and Cl combine to form KCl. The overall net reaction is: $HCl_{(aq)} + KOH_{(aq)} \rightarrow KCL + H_2O$

85- D. selenium

Elements with the highest electrical conductivity are metals, such as aluminum. Metalloids, such as boron and silicon, have intermediate electrical conductivity, lower than that of metals but higher than that of non-metal elements, such as selenium. Non-metals such as selenium have very poor, if any electrical conductivity.

86- C. CO2

Fermentation reactions are usually carried out by biological cells as a form of anaerobic cellular respiration where sugars are variously converted to a variety of alcohols, acids and gases (but never oxygen as a gas), depending on the nature of the specific fermentation reaction. During alcoholic fermentation, yeast cells convert glucose to ethanol and carbon dioxide by the following equation: PC6H12O6 → 2 C2H5OH + 2 CO2.

87- C. natural killer cells

Adaptive immunity consists of two types of immune response, humoral and cell mediated. Natural killer cells may participate in a cell-mediated immune response, but usually they do not. Most of the cell-mediated immune activities involve interactions among foreign or virally infected cells and T-helper, cytotoxic T and B-cells.

88- A. 1 to 1

The Punnett square predicted frequencies of heterozygous offspring from either two heterozygous parents, or one homozygous and one heterozygous parent is 50%. The ration of the two frequencies therefore is 50% to 50% which is the same ratio as 1 to 1 .

89- C. energy and mass

Heat of vaporization is the amount of heat absorbed by either a mass or a molar amount of a substance as it undergoes a phase transition between either a solid or liquid phase to the gas phase. Temperature remains constant during phase transitions so degrees Celsius would not be included in the units for heat of vaporization. Heat is equivalent to energy so the units of heat of vaporization are energy per unit mass or energy per mole. Volume is not relevant to the heat of vaporization of a substance.

90- D. intercellular membrane receptor binding

T-helper cell roles in the immune system usually involve interactions where membrane bound T-cell proteins bind with other membrane bound proteins of other immune system cells, such as B-cells and antigen presenting cell such as macrophages. T-helper cells are not capable of phagocytosis, cell lysis function or circulating antibody production. They are capable of producing antibodies that remain bound to their cell membranes.

91- D. produce fertile offspring

Most species are in competition with other species for the same ecological niche. Genus is a broader taxonomic category than species, therefore more than one species may belong to the same genus. Most species cannot physically interbreed with another species, but some do. An example are the horse and donkey species that can interbreed to create a hybrid offspring, namely the mule. Mules and all other interspecies' offspring are sterile.

92- C. $(2gh)^{1/2}$

The object's gravitational potential energy is equal to mgh. The object's kinetic energy is equal to $\frac{1}{2}(mv^2)$. If all of the potential energy is converted to potential energy this means that $mgh = \frac{1}{2}(mv^2)$. Rearrangement of the equation to solve for v gives $v = (2gh)^{1/2}$

93- A. Iodine; endocrine

Iodine is a critical component of the the thyroid hormones, which are essential to human life. The endocrine system is responsible for synthesis of hormones. Iron is critical for the circulatory system because it is a central component of hemoglobin, but is not directly critical to specific nervous system activity. Copper is a cofactor for several enzymes that catalyze oxidation reduction reactions but copper is not a direct participant in specific digestive functions. Selenium is required by several enzymes that act as antioxidants, but selenium is not directly critical to specific nervous system activity.

94- B. the distance that light travels in a vacuum in 1 year

The speed of light in a vacuum is constant for any observer in the universe. The distance that light would travel in a vacuum in one year is defined as 1 light-year. The speed of light in a vacuum is approximately 3×10^8 m/s. This is approximately 670,000,000 miles per hour or over 5.8 quadrillion miles per year.

95- A. at the junction of the thoracic duct and the superior vena cava
The majority of lymphatic vessels eventually carry lymph fluids toward the major lymphatic vessel, the thoracic duct. The thoracic duct connects to the superior vena cava a short distance before the superior vena cava connects to the right atrium of the heart. The direction of fluid flow at most capillary beds is out of the capillaries and into lymphatic vessels. Lacteals absorb triglycerides from the intestine. They do not absorb lymphatic fluids.

96- B. a biome
Biomes are the broadest subcategory of the ecosphere, which is used to describe the totality of all life and life-sustaining environmental features on earth. Biomes are regions with the same climate and a dominant type of flora and fauna where all of the living species interact to produce a self-sustaining stable network of living organisms. Other examples of biomes include sub-arctic tundra regions that are termed "taiga" and broad grassland regions that are termed "savannahs".

97- C. a molecule
The molecule is the smallest unit of matter as described above. A substance can be virtually any type or combination of matter including mixtures of many different molecules. A crystal has no specific size and can be composed entirely of only one type of elemental atom. An ion can be a molecule, but it can also be an individual atom.

98- D. organisms that carry out photosynthesis
Oxygen is extremely reactive and would rapidly disappear from the atmosphere if it were not being continually replenished by oxygen produced by organisms that convert carbon dioxide and water into carbohydrates and oxygen through the process of photosynthesis. Burning of fossil fuels produces carbon dioxide and consumes atmospheric oxygen. Only a relatively tiny amount of oxygen is produced by lightning hydrolysis. Virtually no oxygen is ever emitted by volcanic eruptions.

99- A. orange wavelength visible light
The wavelengths of visible light beginning with the longest and becoming progressively shorter is: red, orange, yellow, green, blue, indigo and violet. This can be remembered using the mnemonic ROY G. BIV.

100- C. the sternum
The longest bone in the human body is the femur. The ribs may be longer than the humerus, but both are always longer than the sternum, which is commonly call the breastbone.

ADVANCED PRACTICE TEST: SCIENCE

1- B. smooth endoplasmic reticulum does not participate in synthesis of proteins.
Smooth endoplasmic reticulum does not contain ribosomes. Rough endoplasmic reticulum does contain ribosomes. Ribosomes are required to synthesize proteins. Both RER and SER may be involved in the synthesis of products that are destined for transport and secretion out of the cell into the external environment.

2- A. an external cell membrane
An external cell membrane is a feature of all living cells. Many cells such as plant fungi and bacterial

cells also possess at least one outer cell wall, but human and other animal cells do not. Bacterial cells do not possess a nucleus or mitochondria.

3- B. coronal

Coronal refers to an axial plane of the body. The other axial planes are the sagittal and the cross sectional planes. Caudal means nearer to the tail or the posterior part of the body. Ventral means at or nearer to the frontal surface of the body. The term inferior means near to the feet.

4- C. microtubules

Human sperm flagellum are constructed from and internal bundle of microtubules that interact with a microtubule organizing structure at the base of the flagellum. The individual microtubules sequentially slide back and forth within the outer envelope of the flagellum causing a whipping motion that generates a forward motion of the sperm cells. Thick or myosin filaments are critical elements of muscle contraction and actin microfilaments are involved in many functions that require active purposeful movement of cells and within cells but neither are elements of the flagellum of human sperm cells. Intermediate filaments are generally structural elements of the cytoskeletal framework of a cell and do not contribute to the functioning of flagellum of human sperm cells.

5- B. high extracellular matrix volume

Muscle and nerve tissue have high cell volume compared to extracellular matrix volumes. In voluntary muscle the neuromuscular junction is an interface between the terminal endings of axons of neurons and cell membranes of muscle fibrils. Actin filaments are a component of the thin fibers of sarcomeres in voluntary muscle tissue. All muscle cells have electrically excitable membranes that can conduct electrical signals along the surface of muscle outer cellular membranes

6- A. ACG

The nitrogenous base thymine (T) occurs in DNA molecules but not in RNA molecules. The nitrogenous base uracil (U) occurs in RNA molecules but not in DNA molecules. The remaining nitrogenous basis of nucleic acids, adenine (A), cytosine (C) and guanine (G) occur in both RNA and DNA. Codons are DNA 3-base sequences and anticodons are RNA 3-base sequences. Among the choices only choice A has a three base sequence that does not include thymine or uracil. Therefore, this is the only choice that could occur in both an RNA and a DNA sequence.

7- B. acetyl CoA

Acetyl CoA is generated by conversion of pyruvate -an end product of glycolysis and by many other chemical pathways including the metabolism of lipids. It is a starting reactant molecule that enters at the beginning of a Krebs cycle. Two CO_2 molecules, 2 NADH molecules and one $FADH_2$ molecules are among the product molecules generated by each round of a Krebs cycle.

8- C. A polar body is generated

The successful maturation of a human primary follicle into a human secondary follicle occurs in response to the LH peak in the ovulatory cycle. During this maturation phase, the primary oocyte of the primary follicle undergoes a meiotic division resulting in a secondary oocyte and a polar body. The formation of the corpus luteum occurs after the rupture of the secondary follicle and the release of the secondary oocyte. Degeneration of the corpus luteum occurs a few days after ovulation if the secondary oocyte is not fertilized. Increasing estrogen levels trigger an initial luteinizing hormone (LH) peak during an ovulatory cycle but a second peak does not occur during a cycle.

9- D. Leydig; testosterone

Leydig cells of the testes produce testosterone in the male reproductive system. The tunica albuginea is a fibrous outer membrane of the testis and does not directly participate in the production of any particular type of cells. Sertoli cells produce various substances that support the development of sperm cell precursor cells, but they do not produce FSH. Spermatogonia are cells that are progenitors of mature sperm cells. Spermatogonia do not produce LH.

10- A. elbow; knee

The elbow and knee joints are both synovial hinge joints which allow flexion and extension. The elbow joint is a complex hinge joint that also allows the head of the radius to pivot at the articulation of the distal end of the humerus. This allows for additional range of motion in the form of supination and pronation of the lower arm and hand. This additional range of motion is much greater than that allowed by the knee joint. The sacroiliac joint connects the sacrum (triangular bone at the bottom of the spine) with the pelvis (iliac bone that is part of the hip joint) on each side of the lower spine. It is a non-synovial ligamentous joint that has very little range of motion, less than any of the other joints listed in the choices above. The elbow and shoulder joints are both synovial ball-and-socket joints which have a much greater range of motion than hinge joints such as the knee and elbow.

11- D. lung, liver and pancreas

The lung, liver and pancreas are all primarily derived from endoderm. The heart and the kidney are primarily derived from mesoderm. The brain is primarily derived from ectoderm.

12- B. prevention of collapse of alveoli during exhalation

Pulmonary surfactant decreases the surface tension of the fluid layer overlying the internal surfaces of alveoli. The surface tension of fluid layers of a concave surface such as the internal surface of a sphere increases as the radius of sphere decreases. Without pulmonary surfactant the surface tension of the aqueous layer within alveoli would increase as the alveoli deflate during exhalation to a point where the alveoli would completely collapse. This event would prevent reflation of the alveoli on a subsequent inspiratory effort.

13- C. pulmonary artery pressure

A maximal inspiratory effort increases intrathoracic volume by maximally decreasing the convexity of the diaphragm and by lifting the ribs upward and outward through contraction of intercostal muscles (accessory muscles of inspiration). Maximal inspiration increases the volume of lung that is both perfused and ventilated therefore the diffusion of CO_2 into the alveolar airspaces and the diffusion of O_2 out of alveolar airspaces will increase. With additional regions of the lung perfused during maximal inspiration, the total cross sectional area of the pulmonary outflow tract of the heart increases. The total resistance to a fixed amount of blood delivered by the contraction of the right ventricle decreases and the pulmonary artery pressure most likely will decrease rather than increase.

14- B. The right ventricular pressure reaches a minimum value.

Systole is the portion of the cardiac cycle where the ventricles are contracting. The end of systole corresponds with the completion of ventricular contraction. The pressures within ventricle reach a minimum value at the end of their contraction cycles. The aortic valve opens and the mitral valve closes at the beginning of systole. The AV node does not generate electrical impulses but will conduct electrical signals across the AV septum at the beginning of systole.

15- A. the atrioventricular septum

The AV septum tissue is non-conductive and prevents the propagation of electrical signal from the atrium to the ventricles. The exception occurs at The AV node where electrical signals are intercalated discs possess gap junctions that allow electrical signals to propagate through cardiac muscle tissue. Purkinje fibers act as electrical conduction wires within the walls of ventricles.

16- A. a peripheral vein located in the leg

The pulmonary arteries are components of the right cardiovascular circulation system. Blood clots of the pulmonary arteries (thrombotic pulmonary embolisms) must originate from sites within the right heart circulation unless there is an abnormal pathway from the left to the right circulation pathways such as a direct connection between the left and right atrium. Most commonly, thrombotic pulmonary embolisms originate as blood clots in large deep veins of the lower leg. The origins listed in the other choices are all located on the left side of the heart circulation.

17- B. plasma cells

White blood cells or leukocytes include lymphocytes and non-lymphocytes Lymphocytes include T-cells, B-cells and the activated form of B-cells - the plasma cell Eosinophils, basophils, monocytes and polymorphonuclear leucocytes (PMNLs) are all non-lymphocyte lineage white blood cell types.

18- A. HLA class I antigens

The major histocompatibility complex (MHC) class I human leukocyte antigens (HLA) are generally restricted to the cell membranes of dedicated or professional antigen presenting cells of the immune system. T-cells are activated when they bind with a class I molecule and an antigen on the surface of an antigen presenting cell. ABO and Rh factor molecules are generally restricted to red blood cell (RBC) membranes and can be a antigen that is identified as foreign by the immune system. Cadherin class cell adhesion molecules are involved primarily with structural functions related to binding with extracellular matrix molecules.

19- D. lacteals

A common feature of non-glandular epithelial tissues, including the primary cell type of the epithelial lining of the intestines, is polarity. This refers to the separation of structure and functions of the top or apical region of the epithelial cell from lower or basal regions of the cell. Enterocytes at their apical surface (the surface exposed to the contents of the lumen of the intestinal tract) have dense hair like extensions called microvilli. These microvilli vastly increase the surface area of the enterocytes that is exposed to the contents of the lumen of the intestines. This increases the efficiency of the enterocytes ability to absorb water and nutrients from the intestine. Tight junctions and desmosomes knit adjacent enterocytes together at or near their apical surfaces. This creates are relatively impermeable barrier to contents of the intestine, preventing the contents from diffusing between enterocytes. Lacteals are sealed terminals of lymphatic vessels that are located in the cores of intestinal villi that underlie enterocytes. They are responsible for receiving lipids from overlying enterocytes. Theses lipids are derived from lipids absorbed by the enterocytes from the intestine.

20- C. a meal with high simple carbohydrate content

The most common stimulus for the release of the hormone glucagon is low levels of glucose in the bloodstream. The primary effect of glucagon is on the liver, where it induces the liver to break down stored glycogen molecules into glucose molecules. The glucose molecules are secreted into the bloodstream and restore the blood glucose levels toward normal. Conversely, high blood glucose levels have the opposite effect, namely the suppression of the release of glucagon. A meal high in carbohydrates will generally result in high levels of blood glucose, because carbohydrates are composed primarily of glucose monomers. Simple carbohydrates are easily hydrolyzed by enzymes in the digestive tract to glucose molecules which in turn are rapidly absorbed into the circulation. This increases blood glucose levels and consequently tends to suppress glucagon secretion.

21- B. CCK secretion→↑bile secretion→↑fat emulsification

Cholecystokinin release from the duodenum triggers the release of bile from the gallbladder into the duodenal lumen. Bile emulsifies collections of lipids in the duodenum. Somatostatin is a hormone secreted by the duodenum and the pancreas (and anterior pituitary gland) that inhibits HCL secretion and gastrin secretion in the stomach. Secretin is a hormone released by the duodenum that inhibits HCl secretion in the stomach and stimulates the release of bicarbonate by the pancreas.

22- D. potassium ion (K+) diffusion out of a neuron

As the transmembrane potential reaches a positive peak during an action potential, voltage-gated potassium ion channels are activated and K+ ions, which have a higher intracellular concentration compared to extracellular concentration, diffuse out of the cell. This rapidly reverses the peak positive transmembrane potential of the action potential and generates a negative transmembrane potential that is more negative than the normal resting transmembrane potential. This is referred to as hyperpolarization. The effect of hyperpolarization is to cause the local cell membrane to become less likely to generate another action potential. The short period of time that corresponds to the persistence of the hyperpolarization of the local membrane region is called the refractory period of an action potential.

23- A. The release of norepinephrine (NE) into the neuron-myofibril gap of a neuromuscular junction

The choices from A through D summarize the process of contraction that occurs in sarcomeres within a myofibril beginning with the release of a neurotransmitter at a neuromuscular junction. The incorrect step is that the neurotransmitter that is released is not norepinephrine (NE). Acetylcholine (ACh) is the neurotransmitter released at neuromuscular junctions.

24- B. oligodendroglia and astrocytes

Both Schwann cells - in the peripheral nervous system - and oligodendroglia - in the central nervous system - produce myelin sheaths for axons of neurons. Astrocytes contribute to the blood-brain barrier of the central nervous system. Microglia provide metabolic support functions to neurons in the CNC. The axons of neurons can have myelin sheaths, but neurons do not produce myelin themselves.

25- B. the parietal lobes of the cerebral cortex

The primary motor cortices of the parietal lobes contain upper-motor neurons that initial the electrical signal sequence that ultimately triggers voluntary muscle movement. The parietal cortex processes auditory information. Both the basal ganglia and the cerebellum provide additional processing of voluntary muscle signals, but they do not initiate voluntary muscle movement signals.

26- C. inadequate amounts of O_2 delivered to muscle tissue

Lactic acid (lactate) production in muscle tissue results from the anaerobic conversion of pyruvate (predominantly as a product of glycolysis) to lactic acid. This process generates energy but is very inefficient compared to oxidative metabolism of glucose. Inadequate oxygen supplies shift energy production to the anaerobic pathway that generates lactic acid. Additionally, oxygen is required to reduce lactate back to pyruvate. In an oxygen deficient environment, muscle tissue cannot convert lactate back to pyruvate and consequently lactate levels rise within muscle tissue.

27- D. contraction of smooth muscle in the walls of arterioles in voluntary muscle tissue

Parasympathetic nervous system activation produces physiological changes that are associated with resting and digestive functions. Contraction of smooth muscle in the walls of arterioles in voluntary muscle tissue redirects blood flow from voluntary muscles where it can be utilized by the digestive system. Increased sinoatrial node activity results in an increase in heart rate; decreased activity of smooth muscle contractions in the wall of the digestive tract slows peristalsis and inhibits digestive processes. Both of these effects are the opposite one would expect of parasympathetic effects. There are no direct autonomic effects on deep tendon reflexes. These are independent reflex arc consisting of only a sensory receptor cell and one or two neurons in a sequence terminating on a voluntary muscle.

28- C. dendrites

Ligand-gated ion channels respond to the binding of a substance to it membrane receptor. In neurons, these ligands are usually neurotransmitter molecules. The site of release of neurotransmitters by neurons is usually at the synapse of two neurons or at a neuromuscular junction. Neurotransmitters are released by axon terminals of the presynaptic neuron into the synaptic cleft. The neurotransmitters diffuse across to the adjacent membrane region of the postsynaptic neuron. Most often this is the terminal region of a dendrite of the postsynaptic neuron. This is the reason that ligand-gated ion channels are usually most highly concentrated in the dendrites of neurons.

29- B. the seminiferous tubules

The first stage of spermatogenesis occurs in the walls of seminiferous tubules in the testis. Later stages of spermatogenesis occur within the lumen of the convoluted vessels that is the epididymis. The corpus spongiosum is highly vascularized region of the penis that comprises most of the tissue mass of the penis. The seminal vesicles are internal gland of the male reproductive system that provides most of the seminal fluid that nourishes and transports sperm within the genitourinary system. Neither the corpus spongiosum nor the seminal vesicles contain any sperm cells or progenitors of sperm cells.

30- C. medial to the labia minora and inferolateral to the vaginal introitus

The Bartholin's glands or greater vestibular glands are 1 to 2 cm length glands with a terminal ductal orifice located immediately inferolateral (one gland to the left and one to the right) to the vaginal introitus (external entrance). Bartholin's glands secrete mucus which provides lubrication of the vagina.

31- D. gland→dermis→basement membrane→epidermis→external surface of the epidermis

There are two general types of sweat glands located in human integument, apocrine and eccrine sweat glands. The eccrine sweat glands are by far the most numerous and excrete sweat onto the outer surface of the skin. The apocrine sweat glands are located in the lower dermis near the interface with the underlying hypodermal layer of the integument (also called the subcutaneous layer) apocrine sweat gland duct beginning at the origin to the body of the gland must sequentially pass through the overlying region of the dermis and then pass through the basement membrane which separates the dermis from the more superficial epidermis. In the epidermis the duct inserts into a hair follicle and excretes the apocrine glandular oily sweat solution into the space between the keratigenous hair shaft and the outer wall of the hair follicle

32- A. immune - antigen presentation

Langerhans cells are a form of dendritic cell that are located primarily in the epidermis (except for the most superficial layer - the stratum corneum) regions of the epidermis and superficial regions of the dermis. Langerhans cells are antigen presenting cell. In the integument they ingest debris resulting from skin infections and present them on their cell membranes for interaction with other immune system cells.

33- D. connective; energy storage

The hypodermis is the deepest of the three layers of the human integument. It is primarily loose connective tissue with a high content of adipocytes. One of the primary functions of the adipocytes is the storage of fat which serves as an energy reserve for the body. The adipocytes also provide some mechanical cushioning properties to the integument but they allow interstitial fluids and cells to freely pass through the hypodermis. This is the opposite of a barrier function

34- B. melatonin

There are no obvious methods to determine if a hormone is produced by the pituitary other than to memorize which are and which are not. Often this type of question can be answered by recognizing a hormone that is easily identified as the product of another endocrine gland. In this case, melatonin is the only significant hormone produced by the pineal gland and it is not a significant product of any other gland.

35- B. thyroid hormone (T3 and T4)

At the most general level the activation of the sympathetic nervous system induces a high level of overall alertness and priming of the body for high energy activities. Among these effects is an elevated metabolic state. Thyroid hormones in general also induce increased metabolic activity. It is often difficult to distinguish the difference is symptoms between persons with excessive levels of thyroid hormone (hyperthyroidism) and those with extreme activation of the sympathetic nervous system, as occurs with general anxiety disorders, and panic attacks.

36- A. osteoblasts

The non-cellular structural components of bones consist of a matrix of a calcium and phosphorous containing mineral called hydroxyapatite and collagen fibers. Collagen is produced by fibroblasts and the hydroxyapatite that is laid down during bone formation is secreted by osteoblasts. In mature bone, some osteoblasts differentiate into osteocytes' which are sparsely distributed within the center of osteons of bones. Osteocytes secrete small amounts of hydroxyapatite but this is after the bone has been formed. Osteoclasts break down bone matrix - usually during bone remodeling activities. Lamellar bone has well organized arrangements of collagen fibers within the bone matrix. In contrast, woven bone has randomly arranged collagen fibers. Lamellar bone possesses significantly greater mechanical strength compared to woven bone.

37- C. haversian canals

Trabecular or cancellous bone is one of two general types of bone, the other being cortical or hard bone. In contrast to cortical bone, trabecular bone has a porous, irregular structure that forms extensive cavities that contain adipocytes and the progenitor cells of both red blood cells (hematopoietic stem cells). Trabecular bone is diffusely and heavily vascularized. Compact bone is comparatively poorly vascularized, with blood vessels primarily limited to haversian canals. Haversian canals are features of compact bone. Haversian canals are longitudinal passages that contain blood vessels that branch into smaller vessels that provide blood supplies to osteocytes located in lacunae (small hollow spaces) located in the center of osteons (structural subunits) of compact bone.

38- B. temporomandibular joint

Of the four choices, three are completely fused or relatively immobile non-synovial joints. The temporomandibular joint is a highly mobile synovial joint which allows for the chewing motions of the lower jaw (mandible).

39- D. the glomeruli

Arterial blood arrives for filtration by the kidney via the renal artery. The renal artery undergoes several branching to eventually form renal arterioles that extend throughout the renal cortex. Branches of these arterioles form tufts of capillaries that occupy an invagination of Bowman's capsule. Bowman's capsule is a balloon-like expansion of the proximal renal tubule. The combined region of capillary tufts and Bowman's capsule is called a glomerulus. There are over one million glomeruli in the renal cortex. The walls of the capillary tufts are uncharacteristically permeable to water and dissolved solutes such as electrolytes, urea and other substances. The blood pressure inside the capillaries exceeds the pressure of the surrounding extracellular space and of the fluid within the lumen of Bowman's capsule. This pressure gradient drives water and dissolved solutes out of the capillary tufts and into the lumen of Bowman's capsule. The solution that enters the capsule lumen is referred to as a filtrate.

40- C. Increased renal tubule permeability to water

Rational: The effect of antidiuretic hormone on the kidney is to increase the permeability of the renal tubules and collecting ducts to water. This results in the diffusion of water out of the filtrate solution and into the renal medulla where it can be reabsorbed into the circulation by renal capillaries within the renal medulla. This concentrates urine and reduces the loss of additional water from the body that occurs through the excretory system.

41- C. increased secretion of antidiuretic hormone

Osmoreceptors in the hypothalamus and the pituitary gland directly detect plasma osmolality from adjacent capillaries. When plasma osmolality is undesirably high, the osmoreceptors relay this information to the pituitary. The pituitary response is to release antidiuretic hormone (ADH). As discussed in the rationale for question 40, the effect of antidiuretic hormone on the kidney is to increase the permeability of the renal tubules and collecting ducts to water. This results in the diffusion of water out of the filtrate solution and into the renal medulla where it can be reabsorbed into the circulation by renal capillaries within the renal medulla. This concentrates urine and reduces the loss of additional water from the body that occurs through the excretory system.

42- A. an undesirably low plasma sodium ion concentration; renin

The kidney is able to directly detect the sodium ion concentration of plasma within renal arterioles. A response of the kidney to an undesirably low plasma sodium ion concentration (and also to low blood pressure) is the release of the hormone renin. Renin in the bloodstream leads to the production of angiotensin II. Angiotensin II is a potent vasoconstrictor and also stimulates the release of aldosterone from the adrenal gland. The adrenal gland is not part of the kidney - although it does rest upon the superior pole of the kidney. Aldosterone causes the kidney to increase the reabsorption of sodium ion thereby helping to restore plasma ion concentrations to normal levels.

43- A. glucose

Under normal circumstances, glucose molecules that are filtered from the blood into a renal tubule are 100% reabsorbed from the filtrate. This process can be overwhelmed when blood levels of glucose are abnormally high. Glucose in the urine is an abnormal finding and often indicates the presence of type 1 or type 2 diabetes mellitus. The presence of sodium, urea and bicarbonate ion in the urine is normal so clearly these are not completely reabsorbed from renal tubule filtrates

44- C. concentration of urine

The loop of Henle is a U-shaped segment of the renal tubules. It is the mid-portion of the renal tubule - located between the proximal convoluted tubule segment and the distal convoluted tubule segment of the renal tubules. The bottom of the "U" in the loops of Henle are located in the renal medulla. The distal or ascending limb of the loop excretes sodium ion from the tubule into the adjacent interstitium of the medulla. This creates a very high osmolality of the interstitial fluids in the adrenal medulla. The renal collecting tubules pass through the renal medulla on their pathway to the sinuses of the renal pelvis. The permeability of the renal collecting tubules to water can be adjusted by various hormonal influences. The collecting tubules are impermeable to sodium and other solutes. When the tubules are maximally permeable to water, water diffuses out of the tubules into the adrenal medulla interstitium. Since this is a process of diffusion, the maximal concentration of urine or the maximum osmolality of the urine that can be produced is slightly lower than the osmolality of the interstitium of the adrenal medulla. As water diffuses out of the tubule solution, the osmolality of the solution increases. When the osmolality of the two regions are nearly equal the driving force of the diffusion of water disappears as the concentration gradient between the two regions is eliminated.

45- B. decreased glomerular filtration rate (GFR)

The glomerular filtration rate of the kidney is the volume of fluid that is driven out of glomerular capillaries and into the lumen of Bowman's capsule per unit time. This rate is determined by the blood flow rate to the glomerular capillaries and the pressure gradient between blood within glomerular capillaries and the pressure within Bowman's capsule - the greater the pressure gradient the greater the filtration rate. Decreasing blood pressure decreases the magnitude of the pressure gradient and therefore reduces the kidney's glomerular filtration rate.

46- A. increased blood pressure

Angiotensin II is the activated form of angiotensin hormone. Activation of angiotensin begins with the release of the hormone renin from the kidney. Angiotensin II has a direct effect on circulatory vessels causing contraction of smooth muscle cells located in the walls of arteries and veins. This increases the force of the vessel walls on the blood within the vessels resulting in increased blood pressure. Angiotensin II has a direct effect on the proximal tubules to increase Na+ reabsorption. But this is not one of the answer choice options. Angiotensin II also stimulates the release of the hormone aldosterone which has additional effects on the kidney. These effects are indirect effects on the kidney.

47- D. complement proteins

The membrane attack complex is a multiprotein structure that attaches to the exterior cell membrane of disease causing bacteria that have invaded the human body. The MAC punctures the cell membrane allowing contents of the cell to escape and external substances to enter the interior of the cell (cell lysis). This results in the death of the cell. The MAC is formed from activated protein fragments of the complement proteins (the C5b-C6-C7-C8-C9 complement proteins and protein fragments). Complement proteins circulate continuously throughout the body. Over 30 proteins and protein fragments make up the complement system When the either the innate or active immune system is activated, complement proteins may be activated in a sequential cascade, where one activated complement protein or protein fragment catalyzes the activation of the next set of complement proteins. The activation of the complement cascade also produces activated proteins and protein fragment that the phagocytosis of cells and other substances and also act as cell signaling molecules that recruit immune cells to the site of an infection

48- C. chief cells

Chief cells are cells located in the stomach that secrete pepsinogen - a digestive proenzyme. The immune response to viral infection is generally an active immune response requiring the activation of B-cells by T-cells and the differentiation of B-cells -into plasma cells. Plasma cells then produce circulating antibodies that target the specific viral associated antigens. Interferons are circulating proteins that suppress the intracellular replication of viruses and have several other important antiviral functions.

49- D. deactivation of the snake venom toxin molecules by antigen-specific antibody binding

Antivenom to snake venom (and other biological venoms) is created by injecting the venom into lab animals and collecting the animal's blood serum afterwards. The injected animal will generate an active immune response to the venom that includes the production of antibodies that are targeted to antigens present on the venom molecules. In human patients, these antibodies bind to the venom molecules and in the process disrupt the venom's ability to cause injury either by altering the active sites of the venom molecule or by sequestering the venom molecules within antigen-antibody complexes which neutralize the antigen and enhance the clearance of the venom molecules from the body.

50- B. active humoral

The influenza virus contains viral shell proteins of the influenza virus that are recognized upon injection into the body by T-helper cells that have receptors complementary to the injected antigens. The T-cells activate B-cells with complementary antibody capability. Activation induces B-cell differentiation into plasma cells which actively release antigen specific antibodies into the circulation. These antibodies are short lived and will not protect against influenza infection after a few days. The exposure to the vaccine proteins antigens also results in the differentiation of some of the activated B-cells into long-lived memory cell that can generate a much stronger and more rapid antibody response to a subsequent encounter with infectious influenza viral particles. This rapid response is sufficient to prevent the viral particles from infecting significant numbers of cells in the body. The antibody response is part of the active immune response (vs. the innate immune response) and is categorized as the humoral division of the active immune response (vs. the cellular cell-dependent active immune response).

51- B. bone marrow; thymus

All circulating red and white blood cell types of the human body originate from hematopoietic stem cells located in the bone marrow (and a few other regions in some circumstances in some individuals). Immature T-cells then migrate to the thymus early in life. These immature T-cells, as a group, have at least a few T-cells have the ability to respond to almost any possible specific molecular antigen including all of the antigens that are present in the host body. In the thymus, those T-cells that are capable of reacting to host antigens are detected and eliminated. Without this vital selection process, these T-cells would trigger immune system attacks against the body's own cells. This T-cell screening process continues into the early- to mid-teenage years. Afterwards the thymus progressively decreases in size and functionality.

52- B. redness and heat only

The four cardinal signs of localized infection are the result of the effects of various molecules that are generated by injured and infected cells and by immune cells that migrate to the site of infection. The most important of these molecules are histamines and prostaglandins. One of the effects of these molecules is to induce dilation of the local blood vessels - resulting in redness and increased heat due to increased local blood flow. Swelling is due to the accumulation of fluids and other substances that leak from the local blood vessels due to the increased permeability of the vessels induced by the infection-associated molecules. The pain associated with a localized infection is in part indirectly due to vascular permeability since increased swelling can trigger pain receptors. Pain is also a direct effect of the infection-associated molecules.

53- A. type 1 diabetes mellitus

Type 1 diabetes is a disease where the body produces either inadequate amounts of insulin or more commonly no insulin. In diabetes type 1, the immune system attacks the insulin-producing beta cells in the pancreas and destroys them. Cystic fibrosis and sickle cell disease are classic genetic diseases characterized by dysfunctional alleles of specific genes. Peptic ulcer disease is usually a result of chronic infection of the stomach by the bacteria H. pylori. The Nobel Prize in medicine was awarded to the physician who proved this was true.

54- B. antigen→mast cell release of histamine

Seasonal pollen and mold allergies (hay fever) are a type I hypersensitivity reaction. Hypersensitivity reactions are caused by activation of the immune system in response to relatively harmless substances or excessively strong immune responses to relatively minor infectious or toxic chemical exposure. Hay fever is a hypersensitivity to airborne pollen or molds that are otherwise not harmful to the mucosal tissue of the upper airway epithelium. Mast cells are immune response cell that contain large amounts of histamine and other substances that can trigger inflammation processes. Mast cells are located within or just deep to the epithelial tissue of respiratory airways. Pollen or mold antigens that are inhaled subsequently diffuse into upper respiratory epithelial tissue and bind to receptors on mast that are complementary to these antigens. This triggers the release of histamine into the surrounding tissue. The effects of histamine are dilation and increased blood flow in local blood vessels, increased permeability of local blood vessels and direct and indirect chemical irritation of local sensory nerve fibers and adjacent cells within the epithelia tissues. These effects generate the typical signs and symptoms of hay fever including itching, nasal congestion sneezing, watery eyes and increased watery mucous secretion within the upper airways.

55- A. $AA_1 + AA_2 \rightarrow AA_1\text{-}AA_2 + H_2O$

Single chain proteins are linear amino acid polymers that are synthesized by formation of peptide bonds between individual amino acid monomers. Amino acids contain an amine group (-NH2) and a carboxylic acid group (-COOH) bonded to a central carbon atom. Peptide bonds are formed between adjacent amino acids in a polypeptide chain through a dehydration (condensation) reaction of the amine group of one amino acid and the carboxylic acid of an adjacent amino acid. Dehydration reactions produce a one or more H2O molecules as a product of each individual dehydration reaction. Amino acids can form two peptide bond with other amino acids by forming one peptide bond through a dehydration reaction with their carboxylic acid group and the amine group of an adjacent amino acid and a second peptide bond through a dehydration reaction with their amine group and the carboxylic acid group of an adjacent amino acid.

56- A. immune sentinel cell membrane toll-like receptor binding to bacterial pathogen associated molecular patterns (PAMPs)

Infectious bacteria and other infectious agents have several common general patterns of molecular structure called pathogen associated molecular patterns (PAMPs) that are recognized by complementary membrane receptors of macrophages, dendritic cells and other immune surveillance cells in the body. These receptors come in several varieties and as a group are called toll-like receptors. Once the PAMP-toll-like receptor binding occurs, the immune surveillance cells release several types of cell signaling molecules that trigger the various cellular and chemical immune pathway responses to the infectious agent.

57- A. glycerol + 3 fatty acid molecules → triglyceride + 3 H_2O

A triglyceride can be directly synthesized from one glycerol molecule and three fatty acid molecules. A glycerol molecule has three hydroxyl groups (-OH) and fatty acids consist of a hydrocarbon chain (R group) with a terminal carboxylic acid group (-COOH). Each hydroxyl group on the glycerol molecule can undergo a dehydration (condensation) reaction with a carboxylic acid group on a tatty acid molecule. This creates an acyl group (-COO-) that connects the hydrocarbon R group of the former carboxylic acid to one of the three carbons of the former glycerol molecule. When this occurs at all three hydroxyl groups on a glycerol molecule the resulting molecule is a triglyceride. All condensation/dehydration reactions produce H_2O as a product of the reaction. There are three condensation reactions required to produce a triglyceride from one glycerol molecule and three fatty acid molecules so three H_2O molecules are created by this synthesis reaction.

58- D. glucose molecules→cyclic configuration glucose monomers in branching chain polymer molecules

Glycogenesis in the liver - in general - is the formation of branching polymer chain molecules composed of glucose monomers. Most simple sugars, including glucose, can exist in a linear or a cyclic (ring) form. In glycogen, glucose monomers are locked in the cyclic configuration.

59- A. an individual chromatid always consists of one continuous single-strand form of a DNA molecule

DNA molecules in chromosomes are always in the double-strand form. A chromosome may consist of a single chromatid (following metaphase of mitosis and meiosis 2 and before the subsequent interphase stage of the cell cycle) or in the sister chromatid stage. An individual chromatid always consists of one continuous single-strand form of a DNA molecule. Chromosome in the sister-chromatid form have two identical sister chromatids and therefore have two continuous double-strand form DNA molecules.

60- A. failure of separation of the chromosome 21 tetrad form during meiosis 1 division of gametogenesis

Tetrads are paired autologous chromosomes. The tetrad form of chromosome 21 consists of the two copies of chromosome 21 arranged one alongside the other. Tetrad forms of chromosome pairs occur only during the first meiotic division of gametogenesis. Sister chromatid separation occurs only during the 2nd meiotic division of gametogenesis. Failure of separation of the chromosome 21 tetra during gametogenesis could result in a daughter cell with two copies of chromosome 21. If this cell matures to an ovum that is subsequently fertilized by a normal sperm cell (which contains one copy of chromosome 21), the zygote formed by this fertilization will have three copies of chromosome 21. All the progeny cells of subsequent mitotic divisions beginning with the mitotic division of the zygote will also have three copies of chromosome 21. All of the somatic cells in an individual's body are derived from mitotic divisions that began with the zygote. Therefore all somatic cells would have three copies of chromosome 21. Failure of sister chromatid separation would result in a gamete with single-chromatid-form chromosomes of all 22 autosomes except for chromosome 21 which would be a sister-chromatid form. Upon fertilization the resulting zygote would have one sister chromatid form of chromosome 21 from the sperm cell and one sister-chromatid form of chromosome 21 from the ovum. The result of subsequent mitotic divisions beginning with this zygote would be unpredictable but it is difficult to explain how this abnormality could produce progeny cells all of which have three copies of a normal chromosome 21. The condition described in the question actually occurs in humans and is one of the most common congenital chromosome abnormalities. It is known as trisomy 21 or

Down's syndrome.

61- C. A-U

The correct nitrogenous base pairing between two complementary strands of DNA molecules is thymine (T) with adenine (A) and guanine (G) with cytosine (C). During transcription of a strand of a DNA molecule, the complementary strand of an RNA molecule substitutes uracil (U) for T. Therefore there is an additional correct complementary base pairing between a DNA and an RNA molecule, namely A-U. Overall there are three correct base pairings, A-T, G-C and A-U.

62- A. 100% PpQq

This question can be answered by constructing a Punnett square for a dihybrid cross of PPQQ X ppqq. The question is more easily answered by realizing that one parent is PPQQ (homozygous dominant) and the other is ppqq (homozygous recessive) for the two genes. Since every offspring will receive exactly one and only one allele of each gene from each parent, the only possible genetic profile for the two genes in any offspring is PpQq.

63- C. filled valence octets

Both argon and krypton have filled valence s and p orbital and these are the valence octet electrons that are filled for all group VIII elements. After the n=2 electron energy shell level, the correlation between the completion of the valence energy shell and the group VIII elements (the noble gases) is no longer valid. At the third period, there are eight elements. These eight elements, beginning with the group I element sodium (Na), sequentially add electrons to the 3s and then the 3p orbitals. The final element in the third period, the group VIII noble gas argon(Ar) has eight valence electrons - 2 in the 3s orbital and two each in each of the three 3p orbitals. For argon there are also five 3d orbitals available at the n=3 electron energy shell. Argon has no electrons in the 3d orbitals so it does not have a filled n=3 level. Argon is located in the third row of the periodic table. By definition this is the third period of the periodic table. Krypton is in the fourth period of the periodic table. The outer or valence electron shell diameter determines the atomic diameter of atoms. Krypton atoms have s and p valence electrons in the n=4 electron shell. Argon has no electrons in the n=4 electron shell. The n=4 shell is farther from the nucleus than the n=3 shell so krypton has a larger atomic radius than argon.

64- B. two sigma bonds and two pi bonds

To satisfy their respective valence octets, carbon seeks to acquire 4 additional electrons through sharing of electrons through the formation of 4 covalent bonds with other atoms and oxygen seeks to acquire 2 electrons that can be acquired in the form of electron sharing through the formation of two covalent bonds with an atom or atoms. This occurs in the molecule CO_2 where a single central carbon atom forms double bonds with each of two oxygen atoms. Double bonds are formed between two atoms by the formation of one sigma bond and one pi bond.

65- A. lithium fluoride (LiF)

Ionic bonds between cations and anions occur when there is a large difference in ionization energies of the parent neutral atoms of the cations and anions. The greater the difference in these ionization energies the less covalent or "electron sharing" character of the ionic bonds. The analysis is somewhat more complex for MgCl2 and MgCl2 since there are second ionization energies for Mg and Cl, but lithium is the least electronegative of all the atoms in the answer choices and fluorine is the most electronegative so there no doubt that this choice is the one where the largest difference in electronegativities exists.

66- A. sodium

Although the general trend for ionization energies in the periodic table is that ionization energies increase from right to left and decrease from top to bottom, sodium has only one valence electron. The second ionization energy would be the energy required to remove an electron from sodium's filled n=2 electron energy shell. This second ionization would break sodium's filled 2s 2p octet. This would always require a higher second ionization energy than the second ionization energy for any non-octet valence electron.

67- C. $CO_2 + H_2O \rightleftharpoons H_2CO_3$

One of the most important buffer (pH range stabilizer) systems in the human body is the carbon dioxide/H_2O -carbonic acid-bicarbonate ion reactions that occurs primarily within the bloodstream and in the kidney. The reversible reaction sequence is

$CO_2 + H_2O \rightleftharpoons H_2CO_3 \rightleftharpoons HCO_3^- + H^+$

This is also the reaction sequence that is used by the pancreas to produce bicarbonate ion for secretion into the lumen of the duodenum for the neutralization of acidic chyme from the stomach. The enzyme carbonic anhydrase catalyzes the reversible reaction $CO_2 + H_2O \rightleftharpoons H_2CO_3$.

68- D. the phrenic nerves

The phrenic nerves are the nerves that innervate the thoracic diaphragm muscle. Without the function of theses nerves, contraction of the diaphragm is impossible and breathing cannot occur. Obviously this would result in death. The vestibular nerves transmit information from the vestibular system in the inner ear. Dysfunction of these nerves causes vertigo (dizziness) and difficulty maintaining balance, but this is not necessarily a fatal impairment. The median nerves are somatic nerves that innervate the muscles of the arms. Loss of median nerve function results in numbness and paralysis of portions of the arms. This is not a function that is absolutely essential to human life. The sciatic nerves are the major somatic nerves of the lower extremities. Loss of function results in numbness and paralysis of the legs. Again this is not necessarily an essential function for human life.

69- A. bilirubin

Red blood cells have an average lifespan of 120 days in the human body. When red blood cells die the hemoglobin within red blood cells must be broken down or catabolized to products that can be removed from the body or recycled by the body. This breakdown process begins with the conversion of hemoglobin to biliverdin. The second step is the conversion of biliverdin to bilirubin. Bilirubin is subsequently excreted in bile and urine. Uric acid is a breakdown product of purines from DNA. Urea is formed from ammonia (NH_3) which is a breakdown product from the catabolism of individual amino acids. Urea is synthesized by the liver and excreted through the kidneys.

70- D. endergonic forward, spontaneous reverse

For reversible reactions such as the general reaction A + B $\rightleftharpoons$ C +D the convention is that the left to right reaction is the forward reaction and the right to left reaction is the reverse reaction. When it is not explicitly stated that the reaction is specifically the forward or the reverse reaction, it is assumed that the reaction refers to the forward, left to right reaction. If the reaction A + B ⇌ C +D is simply described as an endothermic or exothermic reaction or as an endergonic or exergonic reaction, it is assumed to refer to the forward reaction where A and B are the reactants and C and D are the products. The reverse reaction designations are always the opposite of the forward reactions for the exergonic vs. endergonic designation and the exothermic vs. endothermic designation. Exergonic reactions are always spontaneous reactions. For choice D if the forward reaction is endergonic, the reverse reaction must be exergonic and therefore the reverse reaction is spontaneous. For choice A, not all exergonic reactions are exothermic or heat-producing reactions. For choice B, all endothermic or heat consuming forward reactions are exothermic or heat producing -NOT heat consuming - reverse reactions. For choice C, not all exothermic reactions are exergonic or spontaneous reactions.

71- B. the ration of the substance's liquid-phase density to its solid-phase density is less than 1

Almost all monomolecular substances have a greater density in the solid phase compared to their density in the liquid phase. This correlates with a solid phase density to liquid phase density ratio (density of solid/density of liquid) that is greater than 1. Water is nearly unique in that it is a monomolecular substance that has a higher density in the liquid phase compared to the solid phase. Therefore the ratio of the solid phase density to liquid phase density that is less than 1. This is apparent in everyday life since anyone can observe that ice floats in liquid water. If the solid phase of water (ice) were denser than the liquid phase, ice would sink in liquid water.

72- A. The activation energy for the forward and reverse reactions is equal

The activation energy for a reaction is the amount of energy the reaction must invest to overcome an energy barrier to the reaction. This energy barrier is present in part because the reaction must reach a transition state where the reactants are spatially oriented and electrochemically primed to transform into the products of the reaction. Both the forward and reverse reactions must invest the energy required to achieve this peak energy transition state, but if the forward reaction is exergonic, it produces energy. This energy must also be added to the peak energy value of the transition state for the reverse reaction to occur. The converse is true for endergonic forward reactions. For example if the forward reaction produces 30 kJ per mole of reactant and must overcome a 10 kJ peak activation energy barrier. The activation energy for the reaction is only the 10 kJ transition state barrier. For the reverse reaction. The 30 kJ per mole energy must be expended as well as the additional 10 kJ to attain the peak transition state energy that exists between the right and left side participants in the chemical reaction. In this case the activation energy for the reverse reaction is 30 kJ + 10 kJ =40 kJ per mole.

73- A. increased ventilation rate

The most important buffer (pH range stabilizer) system in the human body is the carbon dioxide/H_2O -carbonic acid-bicarbonate ion reactions that occurs primarily within the bloodstream and in the kidney. The reversible reaction sequence is:

$CO_2 + H_2O ⇌ H_2CO_3 ⇌ HCO_3^- + H^+$

When carbon dioxide is exhaled from the lungs plasma CO_2 concentrations decrease and the reaction is driven toward the left, reducing hydrogen ion concentrations in the plasma and by definition increasing the plasma pH. When the ventilation rate (volume of air exchanged through the lungs per unit time) increases, the amount of CO_2 that diffuses out of the blood stream and into the respiratory airways increases. This lowers CO_2 levels in the blood, and increases plasma pH. Excretion of bicarbonate ion (HCO_3^-) lowers the bicarbonate ion concentration of the plasma and shifts the reaction to the right, producing more hydrogen ion and by definition decreases the plasma pH. Anaerobic respiration produces lactic acid which increases hydrogen ion concentrations in the plasma. Again this by definition decreases PH. Tidal volume is the volume of air exchange during a normal cycle of one inhalation followed by an exhalation. Decreasing tidal volume decreases the amount of air exchanged per breath and this will reduce the rate of CO_2 diffusion from the bloodstream and will decrease plasma pH.

74- C. 2 A(g) + 2 B(g) ⇌ 4 C(s) + D(g)

Within a sealed reaction vessel increasing the volume of the vessel decreases the partial pressures of all of the gas-phase participants in the reaction. This reduces the pressure stress on the reaction and favors the reaction that produces higher amounts of gas- phase products from lower amounts of gas-phase reactants.. In reaction A, the forward reaction produces 3 moles of gas-phase products from 2 moles of gas-phase reactants. In reaction B, the forward reaction produces 2 moles of gas-phase products from 1 mole of gas-phase reactants. In reaction D, the forward reaction produces 3 moles of gas-phase products from 2 moles of gas-phase reactants. All three forward reactions produce greater amounts of gas-phase products than gas-phase reactants and are therefore favored by increasing the volume of the reaction vessel. In reaction C, the forward reaction produces 1 mole of gas-phase products from 4 moles of gas-phase reactants. The reverse reaction of choice C would be favored by increasing the volume of the reaction vessel.

75- B. -2 Celsius to 1 Celsius

All of the temperature changes are increases of three degrees Celsius. Only choice B requires a phase change of H_2O - in this case from the solid to the liquid phase since the melting/freezing point of H_2O at standard temperature and pressure is 0 degrees Celsius. Phase changes require many times more heat energy to convert a given amount of a substance from a lower energy phase to a higher energy phase than is required to raise the same amount of the substance by a single degree in any of the 4 phases of matter.

76- A. (P)(V)/T

The ideal gas equation is $(P)(V)=nRT$

where the container volume = V, the gas pressure = P, n= the number of moles of gas (or another quantitative unit) in the container, R= universal gas constant and T = the temperature of the gas. To determine the proportional relationship of the number moles of gas within the container and the temperature and volume of the container , the ideal gas law can be rearrange to

$$n = (P)(V)/RT$$

Since R is a constant, it can be excluded from the equation and this gives the proportional relationship between n and the pressure volume and temperature of the system.

$n \propto (P)(V)/T$.

The "$\propto$" symbol means "proportional to".

77- A. a solution with a pH = 8

Liquid water has a pH of 7 meaning it has a hydrogen ion (or H_3O+) concentration of 1×10^{-7} moles/liter concentration. Obviously addition of pure water will have on effect on the solution with the pH of 7 since both pure water and the solution have exactly the same hydrogen ion concentration. Since pH is equal to the negative log of the solution's hydrogen ion concentration, the higher the pH value, the lower the hydrogen ion concentration. For water to lower the hydrogen ion concentration of a solution it must increase the hydrogen ion concentration of the solution. Solutions which have a pH less than that of pure water (solutions with a pH less than 7) have a higher hydrogen ion concentration than pure water. The addition of water to these solutions will dilute the hydrogen ion concentration of the solution resulting in a new solution with a higher pH than the original solution. This eliminates choices C and D. Choice A has a pH of 8, and therefore has a hydrogen ion concentration of 1×10^{-8} moles/liter. The hydrogen ion concentration of pure water, (1×10^{-7} moles/liter) is ten time higher than the pH 8 solution. The addition of pure water to this solution must therefore increase the concentration of hydrogen ion in the resultant solution and by definition lower the pH of the resultant solution.

78- D. The combined concentration of the conjugate base A- and conjugate acid B+ in the resultant solution will be greater than the combined concentration of conjugate acid B+ and OH- in the resultant solution

Strong acids (HA) by definition completely dissociate into hydrogen ions (H+) and the conjugate base (A-). Weak bases by definition only partially dissociate into hydroxide ions (OH-) ions (H+) and the conjugate acid (B+) Since the strong acid HA will completely dissociate into A- and H+ The H+ concentration of the solution will be equal to the HA concentration. 0.1 molar or 1x10-1 moles per liter. This is equivalent to a solution pH of 1. Basic aqueous solutions add OH- ions to an aqueous solution solutions and these can combine with H+ ions but less OH- ions add added to the solution because the weak base has an equal initial concentration to the strong acid but it does not completely dissociate so fewer OH- ions are contributed than H+ ions. By definition aqueous solutions with higher concentrations of H+ than OH- are acidic and by definition have a pH less than 7 and therefore choices A and B are incorrect. Since strong acids completely dissociate the concentration of HA in solution is zero. Weak bases do not completely dissociate so there is some BOH in solution therefore choice C is incorrect. For choice D the rational is lengthy but as an exercise one can use similar reasoning to verify that it is correct. This is an information overload type of question that is common in standardized testing. The key is to use a process of elimination since the other three choices are not difficult to exclude with simple one-step logical reasoning.

79- D. The gas molecules in both samples have the same average kinetic energy

The average kinetic energy of a gas particle is directly proportional to the temperature of the gas sample. Kinetic energy (KE) = (½)(mass)(velocity)^2. For choice A, gas molecules with different masses can have the same kinetic energy, as long as the square of their velocities times their masses are equal. The same argument is true for choice B. Choice C is incorrect, the different gas molecules must have the same ration of mass to velocity squared. This is usually not the same as the ratio of mass to velocity ratio. For example an object with a mass of 2 kg and with a velocity of 4 m/s and an object with mass of 2 kg with a velocity of 8 m/s have the same mass to velocity ratio (1kg/(2 m/s) and 2 kg/(4 m/s) are both equal to 1/2 . the mass to velocity squared ratios are 1/2^2 =¼ for the first object and 2/4^2 = 2/16 = 1/8 for the other object

---

80- C. 18 grams of liquid H$_2$O

One mole is defined as the numerical value 6.022 x 10^{23} (Avogadro's number). One mole of any pure monomolecular substance has a mass equal to its molecular weight in gram units. For instance, the molecular weight of H$_2$ is 2 amu. One mole of H$_2$ therefore has a mass of 2 grams. The molecular weight of H$_2$O is 18 AMU so one mole of H$_2$O has a mass of 18 grams. Therefore, choice C is correct. For choice D, the molecular weight of CH$_4$ is 16 AMU so one mole of CH$_4$ has a mass of 16 grams, not 8 grams. For choices A and B, at standard pressure and temperature one mole of ANY gas will occupy a volume of 22.4 liters, not 1 liter (choice A) and not 20 liters (choice B).

81- A. 9.8 pressure units

Pressure is defined as force per unit area. Force is defined as mass times acceleration. The acceleration on the mass of fluid in the contained is the acceleration due to the force of gravity which is 9.8 m/s^2, therefore the force exerted on the bottom surface of the vessel due to the overlying column of liquid is equal to (1 kg)(9.8 m/s^2) = 9.8 newtons. The area of the bottom inside surface of the container is 1 m^2 since pressure is equal to force per unit area The pressure that is experienced at the bottom of the interior of the vessel is 9.8 newtons/1 m^2 = 9.8 pressure units. In this case the pressure units are kg-/m-sec^2. This pressure unit is called a Pascal (Pa). Another unit of pressure the atmosphere (atm) uses only units of height in millimeters of mercury in a barometric pressure tube.

82- D. 10 m/s

The formula for the kinetic energy of an object is
KE = (½)mv^2.

The calculation for the object described is therefore

$500 = (½)(100)(v)^2$
$v^2 = (2)(500)/100$ kg
$v^2 = 10,000/100$ kg
$v^2 = 100$
$v = 10$

The units of velocity are m/s, therefore the correct answer is 10 m/s.

83- B. 3/π density units

Density is defined as mass per unit volume (m/v). The formula for the volume of a sphere is (4/3) π

r^3 where r is the radius of the sphere. The density of sphere is therefore

Density = mass/(4/3)(π r^3)

Density = 4 kg/(4/3)(π)(1 m)^3

Density = 3/ π kg/m^3

Notice that the density units are mass (in kilograms) per volume (in cubic meters).

84- B. 2 amu

The masses of both the proton and the neutron are both 1 amu to three significant figures - 1.007 amu for the proton and 1.008 amu for the neutron. The mass of the proton is thousands of times lower than 1 amu (0.0005 amu). The nearest of the four choices to the sum of the masses of the three subatomic particles to one significant figure is 2 amu.

85- A. helium to hydrogen

Since the atomic number of an element is equal to the number of protons in the nucleus of the elemental atoms and since the nuclear charge of an atom is equal to the number protons in the atom's nucleus, the correct answer will be the choice with the largest ratio of atomic numbers for the pairs of atoms The atomic numbers are usually displayed at the top of the elemental symbol on a periodic table of the elements. You will be provided with a periodic table during administration of the TEAS. The atomic number for helium is 2 and for hydrogen is 1 so the ratio is 2 to 1 for choice A. By similar reasoning choice B ratio is 7 to 6, choice C ratio is 17 to 19 and choice D ratio is 36 to 19. It should be recognized that one need not calculate these ratios but rather to observe that for choices B,C and D the first value of the ratio is clearly not twice the value of the second value of the ratio, therefore none are as large as the 2 to 1 ratio of choice A.

86- C. insulin

Oxytocin triggers the milk let down reflex in nursing mothers and melatonin plays a role in the regulation of sleep wake cycles. There are other effects of both of these hormones but the complete absence of either has no obvious greater threat to life than the well documented fatal consequences of the absence of either insulin or cortisol from the body. While complete lack of cortisol is eventually fatal if untreated over several months. The complete absence of insulin makes the uptake of glucose from the bloodstream by most cells of the body impossible. Within days to a week or two this causes a severe and progressive derangement in the electrolyte and pH levels within the body that is 100% fatal unless insulin is replaced in the bloodstream.

87- A. compact bone

All of the choices above are composed of connective tissue with a high percentage of collagen content. Ligaments, tendons and cartilage are almost exclusively composed of collagen fibers or collagen molecules. Compact bone contains a significant fraction of hydroxyapatite mineral matrix and a comparatively smaller percentage of collagen content.

88- B. keratin

Keratin is a primary structural protein component of human hair and nails. It has predominantly secondary alpha helical structure and supercoiled helical tertiary structure. Most structural fibrous proteins have a helical structure. Testosterone and DNA have virtually no protein content. Testosterone is a steroid hormone. Steroid hormones are synthesized from cholesterol molecules which are lipids. DNA is composed of deoxyribose sugars, phosphate groups and nitrogenous bases. Hemoglobin is composed of four polypeptide chain proteins and has many regions that are helical but overall there is much less helical structure compared to keratin protein.

89- D. R-O-R→ ether; R-COO-R→ aldehyde

All of the functional groups are correctly identified with the exception of the R-COO-R group in choice D. The correct designation for this functional group is an ester, which consists of a carbon atom double-bonded to an oxygen atom (forming a carbonyl group), and single-bonded to another oxygen atom which in turn is single bonded to another carbon atom (in the example this would be a carbon of an R group - a hydrocarbon molecule or molecular segment). Finally, the central or carbonyl carbon is also bonded to a different R group carbon top another carbon of an R group. The correct structure for an aldehyde is R-COH, where the carbon atom is a terminal carbon of an R group and is double-bonded to an oxygen atom and single-bonded to a hydrogen atom.

90- B. A + B ⇋ 2C

When chemical reactions occur in a closed system they proceed toward chemical equilibrium. Chemical equilibrium occurs when there is no free energy to be gained by the reaction proceeding in either a net forward or reverse direction. At equilibrium the concentrations of the reactants and products remains constant and the reaction appears to stop. In reality both the forward and reverse reactions are occurring but at exactly the same rate so there is no apparent change in the concentrations of any of the participants of the reaction.

The equilibrium constant (K_{eq}) for a reversible chemical reaction is the ratio - when the reaction has reached equilibrium - of the product of the concentrations of the products of the forward reaction raised to the power of their stoichiometric coefficients to the product of the concentrations of the products of the forward reaction raised to the power of their stoichiometric coefficients. As with many attempts to explain mathematical relationships in words, this statement is difficult to understand, but the general formula is much clearer. For the general chemical reaction

aA + bB ⇋ cC + dD

When the reaction above reaches equilibrium, the equilibrium constant (Keq) for the reaction is

$$K_{eq} = [C]^c[D]^d /[A]^a[B]^b$$

The bracket symbols such as [A] indicate "the concentration of " whichever participant is identified inside the brackets. The concentration units are usually moles/liter (mol/l)

Let us use the correct answer - answer "B" to illustrate.
The chemical reaction for choice B is

A + B ⇋ 2C

Therefore, the equilibrium constant (Keq) for the reaction is

$K_{eq} = [C]^2/[A][B]$

For choice C the reaction is

$2A + 2B \leftrightharpoons C$

Therefore, the equilibrium constant (Keq) for the reaction is

$K_{eq} = [C]/[A]^2[B]^2$

Notice how the stoichiometric coefficients for each participant are the exponential values for the concentration of the participant in the Keq equation.

The question states that equilibrium the concentrations of all participants are equal. This is usually not true for a particular reaction, but given that in this case it is we can substitute the value x for every participant's equilibrium concentration value (since they are all equal). For choice B

$A + B \leftrightharpoons 2C$

This gives an equilibrium constant (Keq) for the reaction of

$K_{eq} = [C]^2/[A][B]$
$K_{eq} = [x]^2/[x][x]$
$K_{eq} = [x]^2/[x]^2$
$K_{eq} = 1$

There are other stoichiometric values that can also give a $K_{eq} = 1$ for this scenario but none of the other answer choices options will; for example, choice C.

$2A + 2B \leftrightharpoons C$
$K_{eq} = [C]/[A]^2[B]^2$
$K_{eq} = [x]/[x]^2[x]^2$
$K_{eq} = [x]/[x]^4$
$K_{eq} = 1/[x]^3$

It is a lengthy explanation but once the concept is understood it can be applied quickly to similar questions in a test situation.

91- C. subnormal ovarian function

The leading cause of osteoporosis is a lack of certain hormones, particularly estrogen in women and testosterone in men. Menopause is accompanied by lower estrogen levels due to reduced secretion of estrogen by the ovaries and postmenopausal women are at greatly increased risk for osteoporosis. Excess cortisol secretion (hypercortisolism) can cause osteoporosis but cortisol is secreted by the adrenal cortex, not the adrenal medulla. Vitamin D deficiency can increase the risk for osteoporosis but vitamin E deficiency is not associated with increased risk for the condition.

92- A. myocardial infarction → high HDL cholesterol levels

High levels of HDL cholesterol are considered beneficial and are associated with a lower risk of atherosclerosis and coronary artery disease. LDL cholesterol levels are associated with increased risk for myocardial infarction (heart attack). High blood pressure is the other major risk factor for atherosclerosis and the diseases associated with atherosclerosis including stroke. Research indicates ANY amount of exposure to UV light -which occurs with any exposure to sunlight, even normal exposure - increases the risk for malignant melanoma. The spleen is a major lymphatic organ that plays an important role in the defense against infection by certain forms of bacteria. Most notably pneumococcus bacteria that cause pneumococcal pneumonia. Person who have their spleens removed are always administered pneumovax - a vaccine against the most common strains of pneumococcal bacteria that are responsible for bacterial pneumonia.

93- D. X chromosome, recessive

Male color blindness is one of the most common sex-linked abnormalities. The gene is located on the X chromosome. The Y chromosome is essentially an X chromosome that is missing one of the "legs" of the X chromosome. The gene for colorblindness is located on the leg of the X chromosome that is missing in the Y chromosome. Males therefore only have one copy of the gene and will develop the disease if they inherit the recessive form of the gene from their mothers. Females have two copies of the gene since they have two X chromosomes. It is much less likely that they will develop color-blindness because the gene is recessive and therefore the recessive form of the gene must be present on each of the two X chromosomes for the condition to occur.

94- A. vitamin B-12 deficiency

Vitamin B-12 is essential for the maturation of healthy red blood cells. Most forms of anemia (low red blood cell levels) are the result of iron deficiency, usually due to blood loss in menstruating women. Vitamin B-12 deficiency associated anemia cannot be corrected by additional intake of dietary or other sources of iron. One important cause of B-12 deficiency is the lack of production of intrinsic factor by the stomach. Intrinsic factor is required for the intestinal absorption of vitamin B-12 Vitamin. This type of anemia is called pernicious anemia and will not respond to increased oral intake of vitamin B-12. Persons with pernicious anemia require regular intravenous injections of vitamin B-12.

95- D. RNA virus; cytotoxic T-cells (CD8 cells)

The HIV virus is responsible for one of the deadliest pandemics in modern human history - acquired immunodeficiency syndrome (AIDS). The virus is also in part responsible for a revolutionary discovery in biology - that the paradigm that all life progresses from information stored in DNA molecules that is transcribed into RNA molecules and then translated into protein molecules was incorrect This was referred to as the central dogma of living organisms. The HIV virus violated this central dogma. HIV genetic information is stored in RNA molecules. The viral RNA codes for - among other proteins - a reverse transcriptase that transcribes the viral RNA into DNA in HIV infected cells. HIV is therefore categorized as an RNA virus. The most significant target of the HIV virus is human T-helper cells (CD4 T-cells). T-helper cells have an absolutely critical role in the active immune system. HIV infection kills T-helper cells and consequently cripples the body's active immune system. Prior to modern antiviral therapy, HIV infection was nearly 100% fatal.

96- A. partial pressure of arterial O$_2$: pons and medulla oblongata

Specialized structures located in the walls of aorta and the carotid arteries called the aortic and carotid bodies respectively are able to measure the partial pressure of oxygen (PaO$_2$) contained in the arterial blood flowing past these structures. Sensory cells in the carotid and aortic bodies relay this information to the pons and hypothalamus which adjust the ventilation rate of the lungs to adjust and maintain an optimum level of oxygen within the arterial blood. The partial pressure of CO$_2$ is measured directly in the medulla and pons and indirectly as corresponding cerebrospinal fluid pH in the medulla.

97- B. cortisol

Cortisol is the primary glucocorticoid hormone of the human body. It has wide ranging effects on virtually all of the functions of the human body but in particular regulates energy metabolism in the body by stimulating gluconeogenesis, by increasing the breakdown of stored fats into substrates that can used as substrates for new glucose formation and by shifting the usage of amino acids from protein synthesis to pathways that can generate new glucose molecules. In the immune system cortisol participates in a feedback system that limits the inflammatory processes that occur due to activation of the immune system. The name "glucocorticoid" derives from early observations that these hormones were involved in glucose metabolism. In the fasted state, cortisol stimulates several processes that collectively serve to increase and maintain normal concentrations of glucose in blood.

98- D. traits resulting from genes located adjacent to each other on the same chromosome

The law of independent assortment refers to traits that appear to be inherited independent of other traits. Traits due to genes located on separate chromosome will occur in a parental gamete with frequencies that are not linked - in other words the fact that one of the trait genes is present in a parental gamete has no correlation to the probability that the other trait gene will also be present in the same parental gamete other than that the probability is that expected by random chance. Linked genes occur together at frequencies higher than predicted by random chance. When g these genes are located on the same chromosome it is much more likely that they be distributed to the same gamete. This correlation would be 100% if crossing over between homologous chromosomes did not occur during meiosis I of gametogenesis. If one of the genes located on the same chromosome is on a segment of the chromosome that is exchanged for the corresponding segment of the other homologous chromosome by crossing over during meiosis. The two genes would then be on separate chromosomes that could assort independently. The further apart two genes are on a single chromosome the more likely it is that they could be separated by crossing over events. The least likely separation of the two genes due to cross over occurs when the two genes are adjacent to each other on the chromosome. In this case the crossover would have to occur exactly between the two genes.

99- B. the hepatic portal vein

Proteins are absorbed from the intestine in the form of single amino acids and small di- and tripeptides that result from the enzymatic cleavage of protein s by proteolytic enzymes in the small intestines. Theses amino acids and small amino acids segments are absorbed by intestinal enterocyte and then are transported into the hepatic portal vein where they are carried to the liver for further processing. This is the reason that the highest concentrations of free amino acids occur in the hepatic portal vein. Free amino acids are found in lower concentrations in the general circulation, lower on the venous side than the arterial side since arterial blood is the route that transports amino acids to cells. The thoracic duct is a major lymphatic vessel that can have high protein content but not individual amino acid content.

100- B. a fungal infection

"Myco"" is the prefix of "related to organisms of the kingdom fungi; "osis" means "abnormal condition" In the case of an abnormal fungal condition of the human body this is synonymous with fungal infection. Excessive myoglobin levels in the bloodstream occur due to excessive breakdown of muscle tissue resulting in myoglobinemia - myoglobin is a hemoglobin -like molecule found primarily in muscle tissue. The medical term for nearsightedness is myopia.

ADVANCED PRACTICE TEST: MATHEMATICS

1 – C. 7/3

An improper fraction is a fraction whose numerator is greater than its denominator. To change a mixed number to an improper fraction, multiply the whole number (2) times the denominator (3) and add the result to the numerator. Answer C is the correct choice.

---

2 – A. 0.6 x 90

To find 60% of 90, first convert 60% to a decimal by moving the decimal point two places to the left. Then multiply this decimal, 0.6, times 90. Answer A is the correct choice.

---

3 – B. $2\frac{5}{6}$

To convert an improper fraction to a mixed number, divide the numerator by the denominator. In this case, you get 2 with a remainder of 5. 2 becomes the whole number and the remainder is the numerator. Answer B is the correct choice.

---

4 – C. 0.6363…

The ratio 7/11 implies division, so the decimal value can be determined by the long division problem of 7 divided by 11. The long division results in the repeating decimal 0.6363… There may be a simpler method to find this decimal. The ratio 7/11 is the product of 7 times 1/11. The ratio 1/11 is the repeating decimal 0.0909… so multiplying that decimal by 7 is 0.6363... provides the same answer. If it seems like the same amount of effort, remember that every fraction with 11 in the denominator can be determined in the same way. Answer C is the correct choice.

---

5 – A. 0.625

The ratio implies division, so 5/8 can be determined by the long division problem of 5 divided by 8. The long division results in the decimal 0.625. There is a simpler method to find this decimal. The ratio 5/8 is the product of 5 times 1/8. The ratio 1/8 is the decimal 0.125 so multiplying that decimal by 5 is 0.625, which is the same answer. If it seems like the same amount of effort, remember that every fraction with 8 in the denominator can be determined in the same way. Answer A is the correct choice.

---

6 – D. 9/16

The numerator in the correct ratio will be equal to the given decimal times the correct denominator. It is simply a result of cross multiplying. But first, these problems can be greatly simplified if we eliminate incorrect answers.

For example, answers A and B can both be eliminated because they are both less than 0.5 or ½. If you can't see that, then multiply .5 times 15 and .5 times 23. In answer A, .5 times 15 is 7.5 so 7/15 is less than the fractional value of 0.5625. In B, .5 times 23 is 11.5 so 11/23 is less than the fractional value of 0.5625.

Now, evaluating fractional answers this way, you may look at answer C and realize that since 0.6 times 8 equals 4.8. Since 4.8 is less than the numerator and 0.6 is larger than the given decimal value, C can be eliminated. Answer D is the correct choice.

7 – A. 5/16

The numerator in the correct ratio will be equal to the given decimal times the correct denominator. It is simply a result of cross multiplying. But first, the problem can be simplified if we eliminate impossible answers.

For example, answer B can be eliminated because it simplifies to 1/6 which is much less than 0.3125. If you can't see that, then divide 1 by 6 which becomes 0.167.

For answer D, the ratio 9/25 is a simplified form of 36/100 or 0.36. 0.36 is greater than 0.3125, so answer D can be eliminated.

Now, evaluating fractional answers this way, you may eliminate answer C for a very simple reason. 19 times 0.3125 will always leave a value of 5 in the ten-thousandths place because 19 times 5 equals 95. That means the product can never be the whole number 6, so answer C can be eliminated.

The correct answer is D because you have logically eliminated all the other possible choices.

8 – A. 6

If $a = 10$, then $2a = 20$.

Now compute the value of b^2

$b^2 = (b) \bullet (b)$
$b^2 = (-4) \bullet (-4)$
$b^2 = 16$

So now you have:

$$\sqrt{16 + 20} \ or \ \sqrt{36}$$

The square root of 36 is 6. Answer A is the correct choice

---

9 – C. 16

The greatest common factor of two numbers is the largest number that can be divided evenly into both numbers. The simplest way to answer this question is to start with the largest answer (32) and see if it can be divided evenly into 48 and 64. It can't. Now try the next largest answer (16), and you see that it can be divided evenly into 48 and 64. 16 is the correct answer. The other answers are also factors but the largest of them is 16. Answer C is the correct choice

---

10 – D. 21/32

To multiply fractions, multiply the numerators and the denominators. In this case, multiply 3 times 7 and 4 times 8. The answer is $^{21}/_{32}$. Answer D is the correct choice.

---

11 – A. 12

Replace the letters with the numbers they represent and then perform the necessary operations.

$3^2 + 6(0.5)$

$9 + 3 = 12$

Answer A is the correct choice.

---

12 – B. 40

The least common multiple is used when finding the lowest common denominator. The least common multiple is the lowest number that can be divided evenly by both of the other numbers.

Here is a simple method to find the least common multiple of 8 and 10. Write 8 on the left side of your paper. Then add 8 and write the result. Then add another 8 to that number and write the result. Keep going until you have a list that looks something like this:

$$8 \quad 16 \quad 24 \quad 32 \quad 40\ldots$$

This is a partial list of multiples of 8. (If you remember your multiplication tables, these numbers are the column or row that go with 8.)

Now do the same thing with 10.

$$10 \quad 20 \quad 30 \quad 40\ldots$$

This is the partial list of multiples of 10.

Eventually, the numbers will be found in both rows. That smallest common number is the least common multiple. There will always be more multiples that are common to both rows, but the smallest number is the least common multiple.

Answer B is the correct choice

---

13 – C. 17/24

To add 1/3 and 3/8, you must find a common denominator. The simplest way to do this is to multiply the denominators: 3 x 8 = 24. So 24 is a common denominator. (This method will not always give you the <u>lowest</u> common denominator, but in this case it does.)

Once you have found a common denominator, you need to convert both fractions in the problem to equivalent fractions that have that same denominator. To do this, multiply each fraction by an equivalent of 1.

$$1/3 \bullet 8/8 = (8\bullet1) / (8\bullet3) \text{ or } 8/24$$

$$3/8 \bullet 3/3 = (3\bullet3) / (8\bullet3) \text{ or } 9/24.$$
$$8/24 + 9/24 = 17/24$$

Adding 8/24 and 9/24 is the solution to the problem. Answer C is the correct choice.

14 – C. 81

When two numbers with the same sign (both positive or both negative) are multiplied, the answer is a positive number. When two numbers with different signs (one positive and the other negative) are multiplied, the answer is negative. Answer C is the correct choice.

15 – C. 7/10

The simplest way to solve this problem is to convert the fractions to decimals. You do this by dividing the numerators by the denominators.

2/3 = 0.67 and 3/4 = 0.75, so the correct answer is a decimal that falls between these two numbers.

$$3/5 = 0.6 \text{ (too small)}$$
$$4/5 = 0.8 \text{ (too large)}$$
$$7/10 = 0.7 \text{ (correct choice between 0.67 and 0.75}$$
$$5/8 = 0.625 \text{ (too small)}$$

Answer C is the correct choice

16 – D. 7

In this number:

1 is in the thousands place.
2 is in the hundreds place.
3 is in the tens place.
4 is in the ones place
5 is in the tenths place.
6 is in the hundredths place.
7 is in the thousandths place.

Answer D is the correct choice.

---

17 – D. 0.72

The simplest way to answer this question is to convert the fractions to decimals. To convert a fraction to a decimal, divide the numerator (the top number) by the denominator (the bottom number).

$$5/8 = 0.625$$
$$3/5 = 0.6$$
$$2/3 = 0.67$$

So the largest number is 0.72. Answer D is the correct choice.

---

18 – D. 3^4

All positive numbers are larger than the negative numbers, so the possible answers are 42 or 3^4. 3^4 equals 81 (3 ● 3 ● 3 ● 3). Answer D is the correct choice.

---

19 – C. 4.8571, 4.8573, 4.8578, 4.8579

The numbers **4.857 and 4.858** have an unlimited set of numbers between them and the simplest method is to start with another number after the last digit of 4.857. Therefore 4.8571 and 4.8572 are both greater than 4.857 and less than 4.858. Choices A, B, and D, include numbers that are equal to or greater than the larger of the two or less than the two numbers. Only C has all numbers between. Answer C is the correct choice

---

20 – D. 23/5

The numbers 4 and 5 can be multiplied by the denominators in the answer set to see which answers are correct. Only D is correct because 20/5 and 25/5 are the numbers that are less than and greater than the answer 23/5. Answer D is the correct choice.

---

21 – A. 34/5

The numbers 7 and 9 can be multiplied by the denominators in the answer set to see which answers are correct. A is correct because 34/5 is less than 35/5 and 45/5, so it can't be in between. Answer A is the correct choice.

---

22 – A. 9

Begin by subtracting –3 from both sides of the equation. (This is the same as adding +3). Then:

$$\frac{4}{9}X = 4$$

Now to isolate X on one side of the equation, divide both sides by $\frac{4}{9}$. (To divide by a fraction, invert the fraction and multiply.

$$9/4 * 4/9\ X = 4/1*9/4$$

You are left with $x = \dfrac{36}{4} = 9$. Answer A is the correct choice.

---

23 – B. –10

To find the value of q, divide both sides of the equation by –13. When a positive number is divided by a negative number, the answer is negative. Answer B is the correct choice.

---

24 – D. $x = 4$

When you multiply or divide numbers that have the same sign (both positive or both negative), the answer will be positive. When you multiply or divide numbers that have different signs (one positive and the other negative), the answer will be negative. In this case, both numbers have the same sign. Divide as you normally would and remember that the answer will be a positive number. Answer D is the correct choice.

---

25 – C. r = (p - 3) / 2

Begin by subtracting 3 from both sides of the equation. You get:

$p - 3 = 2r$

Now to isolate r on one side of the equation, divide both sides of the equation by 2. You get:

r = (p-3) / 2

Answer C is the correct choice

---

26 – C. $x = 11$

Subtracting a negative number is the same as adding a positive number. So 8 – (–3) is the same as 8 + 3 or 11. Answer C is the correct choice.

---

27 – C. 388

The value can be expanded as 7 x 49 added to 9 x 7 with 18 subtracted from the total. That becomes 343 + 63 -18 with the answer equal to 388. Answer C is the correct choice.

---

28 – B. 42

The value can be expanded as 25 added to 5 x 7 with 18 subtracted from the total. That becomes 25 + 35 -18 with the answer equal to 42. There is another simple way to evaluate this expression. The expression can be rewritten as the product of two expressions (x+9)(x-2). If we substitute 5 for x then this product becomes 14 x 3 which is also 42. Answer B is the correct choice.

---

29 – C. 6804

The simplest way to evaluate this expression is to rewrite it as the product of two expressions. Factoring common factors out the given expression becomes 7x(x + 9). "7x" becomes 189 and x+9 becomes 36. The product of 189 and 36 becomes 6804. In the interest of eliminating incorrect answers, the product of the values in the "ones" column is 6x9 which is 54. The correct answer must end in 4 so the correct answer must be C. Answer C is the correct choice.

---

30 – D. $12

Use the information given to write an equation:

$$530 = 40d + 50$$

When you subtract 50 from both sides of the equation, you get:

$$480 = 40d$$

Divide both sides of the equation by 40.

$12 = d$, Sam's hourly wage

Answer D is the correct choice.

---

31 – A. a number greater than X

When a positive number is divided by a positive number less than 1, the quotient will always be larger than the number being divided. For example, $5 \div 0.5 = 10$. If we solve this as a fraction, $5 \div (1/2)$ is the same as $5 \times (2/1)$ or 10 since dividing by a fraction is the same as multiplying by the reciprocal. Answer A is the correct choice.

---

32 – A. (14 + 24) • 8 • 5

In the correct answer, $(14 + 24) \cdot 8 \cdot 5$, the hourly wages of Amanda and Oscar are first combined, and the total amount is multiplied by 8 hours in a day and five days in a week. One of the other choices, $14 + 24 \cdot 8 \cdot 5$, looks similar to this, but it is incorrect because the hourly wages must be combined before they can be multiplied by 8 and 5. Answer A is the correct choice

---

33 – A. 10

Use the facts you are given to write an equation:
$7 + 4/5n = 15$

First subtract 7 from both side of the equation. You get:
$4/5n = 8$
Now divide both sides of the equation by 4/5. To divide by a fraction, invert the fraction (4/5 becomes 5/4) and multiply:
$(5/4)4/5n = 8 \cdot 5/4$

$n = 40/4$ or 10

Answer A is the correct choice

---

34 – D. 108

The ratio of the two numbers is 7:3. This means that the larger number is 7/10 of 360 and the smaller number is 3/10 of 360.

The larger number is 7 • 360/10 or 7 • 36 or 252
The smaller number is 3 • 360/10 or 3 • 36 or 108

Answer D is the correct choice.

35 – C. $310

The costs of all these items can be expressed in terms of the cost of the ream of paper. Use x to represent the cost of a ream of paper. The flash drive costs three times as much as the ream of paper, so it costs $3x$. The textbook costs three times as much as the flash drive, so it costs $9x$. The printer cartridge costs twice as much as the textbook, so it costs $18x$. So now we have:
$x + 3x + 9x + 18x = 31x$

The ream of paper costs $10, so $31x$, the total cost, is $310. Answer C is the correct choice

36 – D. $\dfrac{(6)(9)}{2}$

The area of a triangle is one-half the product of the base and the height. Choices A and B are incorrect because they add the base and the height instead of multiplying them. Choice C is incorrect because it multiplies the product of the base and the height by 2 instead of dividing it by 2. Answer D is the correct choice.

37 – A. 2,595

The steps in evaluating a mathematical expression must be carried out in a certain order, called the order of operations. These are the steps in order:

Parentheses: The first step is to do any operations in parentheses.
Exponents: Then do any steps that involve exponents
Multiply and Divide: Multiply and divide from left to right
Add and Subtract: Add and subtract from left to right

One way to remember this order is to use this sentence:
Please **E**xcuse **M**y **D**ear **A**unt **S**ally.

To evaluate the expression in this question, follow these steps:

Multiply the numbers in **Parentheses**: 3 • 4 = 12
Apply the **Exponent** 2 to the number in parentheses: $12^2 = 144$
Multiply: 6 • 3 • 144 = 2,592
Add: 2 + 2,592 + 1 = 2,595

Answer A is the correct choice.

38 – B. 3x² - 4x - 15

The words in the problem tell us that the new expression for the length is 3x+5 and the new width is represented by the expression x-3. The area is represented by the product of (3x+5) (x-3). Multiplying the two binomials together with FOIL means that the first term is the product of x and 3x or 3x². All of the multiple choices have the correct first term. However, the last term is the product of 5 and -3, or -15, which means that answer C is an incorrect answer.

Since the middle term is the difference of 5x and -9x, which is -4x, answer B is the only correct answer. If you choose to use the box method to solve these products, you will see the same results and the same factors. Answer B is the correct choice.

39 – C. 14x² +13x + 3

The words in the problem tell us that the new expression for the base is 4x+2 and the new height is represented by the expression 7x+3. The area is represented by the product of 1/2(4x+2) (7x+3). Multiplying the two binomials together with FOIL means that the first term is the product of 4x and 7x and ½ or 14x².

However, the last term is the product of 2 and 3 and 1/2, or 3, which means that answer A is an incorrect answer.

The middle term is ½ the sum of 14x and 12x which is 26/2 x or 13x. Therefore answer C is the only correct answer.

40 – B. 19,098 kg m/s

Momentum is defined as the product of mass times velocity. The conversion of 55 km/hr to meters per second means multiplying by one thousand and dividing by 3600. (seconds per hour). That value,15.28, must be multiplied by the 1,250 kg mass. That answer is 19,098 kg m/s. Answer B is the correct choice.

41 – A. $33,500

Janet has a total of $105,000 in her accounts. 70% of that amount, her goal for her stock investments, is $73,500. To reach that goal, she would have to move $33,500 from bonds to stocks. Answer A is the correct choice.

42 – A. $52,000

Convert 15% to a decimal by moving the decimal point two places to the left: 15% = 0.15. Using x to represent Brian's gross salary, you can write this equation:

$$0.15\,x = \$7,800$$

To solve for x, divide both sides of the equation by 0.15. $7,800 divided by 0.15 is $52,000. Answer A is the correct choice.

43 – C. 20

To solve this problem, first convert 45% to a decimal by moving the decimal point two place to the left: 45% = .45. Use x to represent the total number of students in the class. Then: $.45x = 9$

Solve for x by dividing both sides of the equation by .45. 9 divided by .45 is 20. Answer C is the correct choice.

44 – B. 515
Marisol scored higher than 78% of the students who took the test. Convert 78% to a decimal by moving the decimal point two places to the left: 78% = .78. Now multiply .78 times the number of students who took the test:

.78 x 660 = 514.8 or 515 students (whole number answers)

Answer B is the correct choice.

45 – D. 130,500
The population of Mariposa County in 2015 was 90% of its population in 2010. Convert 90% to a decimal by moving the decimal point two places to the left: 90% = .90. Now multiply .90 times 145,000, the population in 2010.

.90 • 145,000 = 130,500

Answer D is the correct choice.

46 – A. 20
Alicia must have a score of 75% on a test with 80 questions. To find how many questions she must answer correctly, first convert 75% to a decimal by moving the decimal point two places the left: 75% = .75. Now multiply.75 times 80:

.75 • 80 = 60.

Alicia must answer 60 questions correctly, but the question asks how many questions can she miss. If she must answer 60 correctly, then she can miss 20. Answer A is the correct choice.

47 – C. $300
If the phone was on sale at 30% off, the sale price was 70% of the original price. So

$210 = 70% of x

where x is the original price of the phone. When you convert 70% to a decimal, you get:

$210 = .70 • x$

To isolate x on one side of the equation, divide both sides of the equation by .70. You find that $x =$ $300. Answer C is the correct choice

---

48 – A. 84

First, find the number of girls in the class. Convert 52% to a decimal by moving the decimal point two places to the left:

52% = .52

Then multiply .52 times the number of students in the class:

.52 • 350 = 182

182 – 98 = 84

Of the 182 girls, 98 plan to go to college, so a total of 84 do not plan to go to college. Answer A is the correct choice

---

49 – C. 12%

To find the percent increase, you first need to know the amount of the increase. Enrollment went from 3,450 in 2010 to 3,864 in 2015. This is an increase of 414. Now, to find the percent of the increase, divide the amount of the increase by the original amount:

414 ÷ 3,450 = 0.12

To convert a decimal to a percent, move the decimal point two places to the right:

0.12 = 12%

When a question asks for the percent increase or decrease, divide the amount of the increase or decrease by the original value. Answer C is the correct choice.

---

50 – D. 14 pounds 14 ounces

When rounding measurements to the whole number value, the measurement is usually rounded up to the next larger whole number if that measurement is halfway or closer to the next higher value. In this case, since there 16 ounces in a pound, D is the correct answer.

---

51 – C. 7,514,635.8239

When rounding a number to a given place value, the next lower place value is used to determine if the number is rounded up or down. The rounded value has its last significant digit in that place. Answer C has a number 9 in the ten thousandths place. Notice the difference between ten-thousands and ten-thousandths. Answer A is rounded to the ten-thousands place!

---

52 – C. 7.15 cc's

When rounding a measurement, the value includes a precision of plus or minus half of the smallest increment measured. The lines on the cylinder would have the values of 7.00, 7.10, 7.20, or each tenth of a cc. The actual value of the meniscus that reads between tenths would be 7.15 cc. Answer C has a number with the correct precision.

53 – C. 4 men for 1 day

When estimating, it is helpful to round before estimating. The summary of this problems solution includes a rate of 200 pounds per hour (15 minute each). Two and one-half tons is 5000 pounds. 5000 pounds divided by 200 pounds per hour means 25 hours of labor is required. Answer C is the best estimate of 25 hours of labor (32). Answer A is 800 hours, B is 16 hours, and D is 200 hours.

54 – B. 40 minutes

When estimating this answer, the basic formula of distance equal to rate multiplied by time applies. So the time required for the trip is the distance divided by the rate. 18 miles divide by ¾ (45 minutes is ¾ of an hour), is 24 miles per hour. The new rate would be 29 miles per hour (increase of 5). 18 divided by 29 is about 60% of an hour or close to 40 minutes. 30 minutes is a close answer, but that is only possible if the rate is 36 miles per hour! Estimating may require that you eliminate answers that are close to the correct answer. Answer B is the correct choice

55 – C. 70 seconds per m/c; 35 seconds per t/f

An estimate often means that you will need to check possible answers to see if they are correct. In this example, the basic assumption is that the time for m/c problems will be twice the value for the t/f. Trying one minute for m/c and one half minute for t/f comes out to 35 minutes. So answer B is not correct. The next closest one is answer C which comes out to 1400 seconds and 1050 seconds for the total 2450 seconds. That is close to the allowable 2700 seconds (45 minutes). If you try answer D, the total comes out to 1600 plus 1200 or a total of 2800 seconds. That's more than the allowable total of 2700. Answer C is the correct choice.

56 – B. twice as fast

When estimating this answer, the formula of distance equal to rate multiplied by time applies. So the speed required for the trip is the distance divided by the time. In this example 10 minutes late means half the amount of time. Dividing by one-half means that the rate must be doubled. Answer B is the correct choice.

57 – D. 1,000,000

The number of square units in this square meter is determined by 1000 rows of 1000 squares of 1 millimeter square units each. 1000 multiplied by 1000 is 1,000,000 units. Answer D is the correct choice.

58 – B. Serena is 7, Tom is 4

Use S to represent Serena's age. Tom is 3 years younger than Serena, so his age is S–3. In 4 years, Tom will be twice as old as Serena was 3 years ago. So you can write this equation:

Tom + 4 = 2(Serena – 3)

Now substitute S for Serena and S–3 for Tom.

(S–3) + 4 = 2(S–3)

Simplify the equation.

S + 1 = 2S – 6

Subtract S from both sides of the equation:

1 = S – 6

Add 6 to both sides of the equation:

7 = S. Serena's age

4 = S-3, Tom's age
Answer B is the correct choice.

---

59 – A. 16 gallons
Amy drives her car until the gas tank is 1/8 full. This means that it is 7/8 empty. She fills it by adding 14 gallons. In other words, 14 gallons is 7/8 of the tank's capacity. Draw a simple diagram to represent the gas tank.

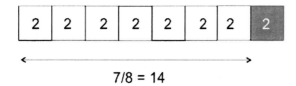

You can see that each eighth of the tank is 2 gallons. So the capacity of the tank is 2 x 8 or 16. Answer A is the correct choice.

---

60 – B. 4.5 inches
The length of the larger rectangle is 12 inches and the length of the smaller rectangle is 8 inches. So the length of the larger rectangle is 1.5 times the length of the smaller rectangle. Since the rectangles are proportional, the width of the larger rectangle must be 1.5 times the width of the smaller rectangle.

1.5 • 3 inches = 4.5 inches

Answer B is the correct choice.

---

61 – C. 32 square inches

The perimeter of the rectangle is 24 inches. This means that the length plus the width must equal half of 24, or 12 inches. The ratio of length to width is 2:1, so the length is 2/3 of 12 and the width is 1/3 of 12. The length is 8 inches and the width is 4 inches. The area (length times width) is 32 square inches. Answer C is the correct choice.

62 – B. 16 feet tall

The ratio of the shadow length and the actual height is a constant determined by the sun. The ratios that apply are tree height / 27 equals 40 / 68. We solve these ratios by multiplying 27 times 40 divided by 67. The correct answer is B.

63 – C. Half a day

The rate for the room is 2.5 man-days per room. The students can apply 5 man-days in one day. One half of a day (answer C) is the required amount of time.

64 – D. 22 gallons

The rate is defined by 23 miles per gallon. The distance divided by the rate is about 21.7 gallons. Answer D is the correct choice.

65 – D. 2.5 hours

The rate is defined by 500 miles per 8.5 hours. That rate means that 140 more miles will require about 2.38 hours (cross multiply 140 • 8.5 and divide by 500). Answer D is the correct choice.

66 – D. 432

Each machine can produce 12 parts per minute (96 ÷ 8). Multiply 12 times 12 (12 machines) times 3 (minutes). Answer D is the correct choice.

67 – D. 3,105

The ratio of female to male students is exactly 5 to 4, so 5/9 of the students are female and 4/9 of the students are male. This means that the total number of students must be evenly divisible by 9, and 3,105 is the only answer that fits this requirement. Answer D is the correct choice.

68 – D. 80

If we call the smaller number x, then the larger number is $5x$. The sum of the two numbers is 480, so:

$x + 5x = 480$

$6x = 480$

$x = 80$

Answer D is the correct choice.

69 – A. $144

When one person dropped out of the arrangement, the cost for the other three went up by $12 per person, for a total of $36. This means that each person's share was originally $36. There were four people in the original arrangement, so the cost of the gift was 4 x $36 or $144.

Let 4x equal the original cost of the gift. If the number of shares decreases to 3 then the total cost is $3(x+12)$. Then those expressions must be equal, so :

$$4x = 3(x+12)$$
$$4x = 3x + 36$$

Subtracting 3x from both sides:

$$X = 36$$

Then the original price of the gift is 4 time 36 of $144. Answer A is the correct choice.

70 – A. 11

If Charles wrote an average of 7 pages per day for four days, he wrote a total of 28 pages. He wrote a total of 17 pages on the first three days, so he must have written 11 pages on the fourth day. Answer A is the correct choice.

71 – B. 2.4 lbs. per week

Six months is half of a year and a year is 52 weeks. The rate will be determined by dividing the total amount by 26 weeks. The rate is therefore 63/26 or about 2.4 pounds per week. Answer B is the correct choice.

72 – A. $12.38 per week

Seven months out of a year is (52 • 7) / 12 weeks. The rate will be determined by dividing the total amount by 30.3 weeks. The rate is therefore $375/ 30.3 weeks or about $12.38 per week. Answer A is the correct choice.

73 – D. 9 months

$3995 divided by $450 per month will provide an answer in months. Numerically the value of that ratio is about 8.88. Since that partial month can't be used, it means that a full nine months will be required to get the full amount. Answer D is the correct choice.

74 – B. 6 months

The difference between the offer and your asking price is $1790 – $1450 or $340. Dividing that value by the monthly decrease equals 340/55 or about 6.18 months. Rounding that value to 6 months, you can now evaluate the acceptability of the reduced offer. Since the partial month can be used as part of your decision process, rounding down to the six months is somewhat a judgment for the seller on the value of the money compared to the value of the car. Answer B is the correct choice.

75 – B. $X \cdot Y = X + Y + 6$

The product of the two numbers is X times Y or X • Y. Therefore,
X • Y equals the sum of the two numbers (X + Y) plus 6. Answer B is the correct choice.

76 – C. 5

Use x to represent the number of women on the board. Then the number of men is $x + 3$. So:
$x + (x + 3) = 2x + 3 = 13$

To isolate $2x$ on one side of the equation, subtract 3 from both sides.

$2x = 10$

$x = 5$

Answer B is the correct choice.

---

77 – B. 65

The average of 25, 35, and 120 is 60. 60 is 10 more than the average of the second set of numbers, so the average of the second set of numbers must be 50. The three numbers in the second set of numbers must add up to 150. Subtract 40 and 45 from 150 to get the answer of 65. Answer B is the correct choice.

---

78 – B. 70

Try each of the answers to see if it fits the requirements in the question.

The numbers divisible by both 5 and 7 are 35, 70, 105, 140, 175…

The multiples of 6 are 6, 12, 18, 24, 30, 36, 42, 48, 54, 60, 66, 72, 78…

Since 70 – 66 = 4; the correct number is 70. Answer B is the correct choice

---

79 – C. 16

There are 9 times as many female nurses as male nurses. To find the number of male nurses, divide the number of female nurses by 9: $144 \div 9 = 16$. Answer C is the correct choice

---

80 – A. 10%

First find the total number of patients admitted to the ER by adding the number admitted for all the reasons given in the question. A total of 120 patients were admitted. To find the percent that were admitted for respiratory problems, divide the number admitted for respiratory problems by the total number admitted:

$12 \div 120 = .10$

Convert this decimal to percent by moving the decimal point two places to the right: $.10 = 10\%$. When you are asked what percent of a total is a certain part, divide the part by the whole. Answer A is the correct choice

---

81 – C. 15 miles

Rebecca's commute is shorter than Alan's but longer than Bob's. Alan's commute is 18 miles and Bob's is 14 miles, so Rebecca's must be longer than 14 but shorter than 18. Neither 14 nor 18 is correct since the distances cannot be equal to either of the examples. So 15 is the only correct answer. Answer C is the correct choice

---

82 – B. 32 diet, 80 regular

If the owner sells 2 diet sodas for every 5 regular sodas, then $^2/_7$ of the sodas sold are diet and $^5/_7$ are regular. Multiply these fractions times the total number of sodas sold:

$^2/_7 \times 112 = 32$

$^5/_7$ x 112 = 80

Remember: when multiplying a fraction times a whole number, it is usually simpler to divide by the denominator first and then multiply by the numerator. Answer B is the correct choice

---

83 – B. The Bulldogs will definitely not be in the playoffs.

The Rangers are playing the Statesmen in the final game, so one of these teams will finish with a record of eleven wins and two losses. Even if the Bulldogs win their game, their final record will be ten wins and three losses. So the Bulldogs will not be in the playoffs. Answer B is the correct choice

---

84 – D. 3,105

The ratio of female to male students is exactly 5 to 4, so 5/9 of the students are female and 4/9 of the students are male. This means that the total number of students must be evenly divisible by 9, and 3,105 is the only answer that fits this requirement. Answer D is the correct choice

---

85 – B. y = –2/3x + 2

The formula for a linear equation is y = mx +b. m is the slope of the line to be graphed and b is the y-intercept, the point where the line meets the y axis.

The slope of the line in this graph is negative because it is moving downward from left to right. So the number before the x will be negative. Answers A and D cannot be correct answers. The slope of the line is expressed as $\frac{rise}{run}$. The slope of this line is –2/3 because it crosses the y axis at 2 and the x axis at 3. The y-intercept, the point where the line crosses the y axis, is 2. The correct equation must be y = $–^2/_3$x + 2. Answer B is the correct choice

---

86 – D. 1

If the y intercept of the line on this graph was reduced by 1, the line would cross the y axis at 2. The slope of a line is defined as $\frac{rise}{run}$. You might also describe the slope of a line as "the change in y over the change in x". If the y intercept was changed to 2, the slope of the line would be 2/2 or 1. The slope of this line is positive because it is moving upward from left to right. Answer D is the correct choice

---

87 – C. ß ß ß ß ß ß ß ß ß ß ß ß ß ß ß/2

If the figures are valued at $450, then dividing $6500 by $450 is 14.44 . C has 14.5 figures which is closest to $6500. Answer C is the correct choice.

---

88 – D. June

To find the median in a series of numbers, arrange the numbers in order from smallest to largest. The number in the center, 92 in this case, is the median. Answer D is the correct choice

---

89 – D. 150 pounds

The average weight of the five friends is 180 pounds, so the total weight of all five is 5 times 180 or 900 pounds. Add the weights of Al, Bob, Carl, and Dave. Together they weigh 750 pounds. Subtract 750 from 900 to find Ed's weight of 150 pounds. Answer D is the correct choice

90 – B. 4

The mode is the number that appears "most often" in a set of numbers. Since 4 appears three times, it is the "Mode". Answer B is the correct choice

91 – C. 78

To find the median in a series of numbers, arrange the numbers in order from smallest to largest:

69, 73, 78, 80, 100

The number in the center is the median. Answer C is the correct choice

NOTE: If there is an even number of values in the series, for example: 34, 46, 52, 54, 67, 81

then the median will be the average of the two numbers in the center. In this example, the median will be 53, the average of 52 and 54. Remember: the median is not the same as the average. Answer C is the correct choice.

92 – D. 102

To find the mean or average, total all the values and divide by the number of values in the sample. In this example there will be 10 grades with an average of 93 points for a total of 930 points. Subtracting the total of points already scored, there are 204 points which are needed to maintain the average. 204 points divided by 2 grades is 102 points per grade. Answer D is the correct choice.

93 – D. 26.5

To find the y-intercept, the patterns in the table must be extended until the x value of the table is equal to 0. Extending the data table to the left means the next two data entries will be 1 and -1. The next two y entries will be 25 and 28. Since 0 is midway between 1 and -1, the y-intercept is midway between 25 and 28. The correct value is 26.5. Answer D is the correct choice.

94 – D. $y = 2x + 7$

The simplest way to answer this question is to see which of the equations would work for all the values of x and y in the table.

Choices A and D would work when x = 0 and y = 7, but A would not work for any other values of x and y.

Choice B would work when x = 3 and y = 13, but it would not work for any other values of x and y.

Choice C would not work for any of the values of x and y.

Only choice D would be correct for each ordered pair in the table

---

95 – D. *y* axis with weight and x axis with date

The data recorded on a "daily" basis implies that the independent data is the time or date of the test. Independent data is normally recorded on the "x-axis". Answers A and D are the two possible correct choices. Since the "weight" is the selected data to be recorded, Answer D is the correct choice.

---

96 – B. Days are the independent variable

The weather data reported on a "daily" basis implies that the temperature data is independent. Since time or date is normally the independent data. Answer B is the correct choice.

---

97 – B. negative covariation

The patient's weight data in this problem is a decreasing value in relation to time. Decreasing as a function of increasing x values is the definition of negative covariation. Answer B is the correct choice.

---

98 – C. 7

The perimeter of the rectangle is 28: 8 + 8 + 6 + 6. If the perimeter of a square is 28, each side is 7. Answer C is the correct choice.

---

99 – C. 2,3,4

The two shorter sides of a triangle must always add up to a value greater than the longest side. Answer C is the correct choice.

---

100 – D. 64

A diagram of the larger square, could be made with 8 rows of 8 smaller squares, so you can make a total of 64 squares. Answer D is the correct choice.

---

101 – A. 64 ft.

We know the dimensions of the left side and the top side of this figure, but how can we find the dimensions of the other sides? Look at the two horizontal lines on the bottom of the figure. We know that together they are as long as the top side of the figure, so together they must total 18 ft. Similarly, the two vertical lines on the right side of the figure, must be as long as the left side of the figure and together they must be 14 ft. So now we know that the perimeter of the figure is 14 + 18 + 14 + 18 or 32 +32 =64. Answer A is the correct choice.

---

102 – B. 32 inches

The radius of a circle is one-half the diameter, so the diameter of this circle is 8 inches. The diameter is a line passing through the center of a circle and joining two points on its circumference. If you study this figure, you can see that the diameter of the circle is the same as the length of each side of the square. The diameter is 8 inches, so the perimeter of the square is 32 inches (8+ 8 + 8 + 8). Answer B is the correct choice.

---

103 – A. length = 12, width = 4

Use *w* to represent the width of the rectangle. The length is three times the width, so the length is $3w$. The area of the rectangle is the length times the width, so the area is $w \cdot 3w$, or $3w^2$.

$3w^2 = 48$

Divide both sides of the equation by 3. You get:

$w^2 = 16$

So the width of the rectangle is 4 and the length of the rectangle is 12. Answer A is the correct choice.

___

104 – B. 10 miles

If you made a simple map with these three cities, it would look like this:

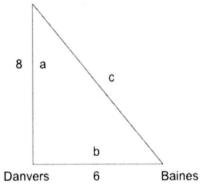

Carson

8 | a

c

b

Danvers   6   Baines

This is a right triangle. The longest side of a right triangle is called the hypotenuse. The two legs of the triangle are labeled *a* and *b*. The hypotenuse is labeled *c*. You can find the length of the hypotenuse (the distance between Caron and Baines) by using this equation:

$a^2 + b^2 = c^2$

In this case, the equation would be:

$8^2 + 6^2 = c^2$

or

$64 + 36 = c^2$

$100 = c^2$

To find *c*, find which number times itself equals 100? The answer is 10.

Answer B is the correct choice.

___

105 – B. 3,024 cubic inches

The formula for the volume of a rectangular solid is length x width x height. So the volume of this box is:

18 x 12 x 14 = 3,024 cubic inches

Answer B is the correct choice.

---

106 – B. 6.5 x 10^{-3}

Make a list of the negative powers of 10:

10^{-2} = 1/100 = 0.01
10^{-3} = 1/1000 = 0.001
10^{-4} = 1/10000 = 0.0001
10^{-5} = 1/100000 = 0.00001

Now multiply each of these numbers by 6.5 to see which one gives you 0.0065. The decimal must be moved 3 places to the left from 6.5 to 0.0065. Answer B is the correct choice.

---

107 – D. 6096

Twenty feet multiplied by twelve inches per foot multiplied by 25.4 millimeters per inch gives a value of 6096 millimeters. Answer D is the correct choice.

---

108 – A. 9.7 millimeters

The square base that is 4 inches on a side has an area of 4•4•2.54•2.54 or about 103 square centimeters. One hundred cubic centimeters divided by 103 square centimeters is approximately 0.97 centimeters or about 9.7 millimeters. Answer A is the correct choice.

---

109 – C. 6.1 cubic inches

One inch is 2.54 centimeters. To convert centimeters to inches, divide by 2.54. Since a cubic centimeter is a centimeter times itself 3 times, to convert we divide by 2.54 three times. 100/2.54/2.54/2.54 equals about 6.1 cubic inches. Answer C is the correct choice.

---

110 – A. 0.00075 kg

Twenty-five milligrams multiplied by 30 capsules is 750 milligrams. Dividing by 1000 is .75 grams. Dividing by 1000 again gives the answer in kilograms.

Answer A is the correct choice.

INTERMEDIATE PRACTICE TEST: ENGLISH

1. A. affected; effect; ought

Since a verb is needed in the first blank, "affected" not "effected" (a noun) will work; but the noun "effect" is correct in the second blank. "ought", meaning "should" correctly completes the sentence, indicating he should not drive. "aught", meaning zero, or nothing, or none, does not make sense in this context.

2. **C. Hiking along the trail, we were assailed by the chirping of birds, which made our nature walk hardly the peaceful exercise we had wanted.**

Who was hiking along the trail? "we" were, so only option C works. The other options are dangling participles: in option b, the birds were not attempting to hike, so that doesn't make sense; in option a, again, the birds were hiking along the trail, so that makes no sense; option d is just poorly constructed and makes the meaning overall unclear.

3. **D. processed**

"Processed" modifies "food products" so that is the adjective; "really" is an adverb modifying the adjective "serious"; "challenge" is a noun, which is a person, place or thing; "consume" is a verb, a word that shows action.

4. **B. My husband and I attended my daughter's dance recital and were very proud when she received an award.**

The most clear and concise sentence is option b; all the information is included, it is presented logically, it flows smoothly off the tongue, and it is not overly wordy.

5. **D. Since the concert ended very late, I fell asleep in the backseat during the car ride home.**

Option d is correct. "Since the concert ended very late" is a dependent clause which explains why "I fell asleep…"; since they are dependent, the only proper way to link them is with a comma.

6. **D. they're**

This question asks you make pronoun and antecedent agree; in this sentence the antecedent is "negotiations"; since this is a plural noun, the pronoun must also be plural, but the blank is also missing a verb. The only option with a plural pronoun and a verb is the contraction "they're".

7. **A. is**

"Group", a singular noun, is the subject of the sentence, so a singular verb is needed. Also needed is a present tense helping verb for "looking forward". The only option that satisfies both is "is".

8. **C. Exclamatory**

An exclamatory sentence is a type of sentence that expresses strong feelings by making an exclamation. Therefore, the above sentence is an exclamatory sentence.

9. **A. Irregardless**

"Irregardless" is incorrect as it is a double-negative: the suffix "less" already indicates a lack of regard, so the addition of the negative "ir" before the correct word, *regardless,* is unnecessary.

10. **C. Between you and me, I brought back fewer books from my dorm room than I needed to study for my exam.**

"Brought" is the correct past tense form of *bring*; "fewer" is the correct word to describe an exact number of items, whereas "less" is used to refer to an amount of something that cannot be exactly counted, like sand or air or water; and "than" is the correct spelling of the word that shows a comparison between two things.

11. **D. us; was**

Words that follow prepositions are considered to be in the objective case, therefore "us" is the correct word here; "Neither", a single pronoun, is the subject of the sentence, so a singular verb, "was" is needed to properly complete it.

12. **C. books**

A noun is a person, place or thing. While a "library" is usually used as a noun to denote a place where people can go to borrow books, or look up information, in this sentence it is used as an adjective to modify "books", which is the only true noun in the sentence.

13. A. Mary and Samantha ran and skipped and hopped their way home from school every day.

A *simple sentence* is one which has *one subject and one verb*, though both the subject and verb can be compound. In this case, option a is a simple sentence, with the one subject being compound ("Mary and Samantha") and the one verb also being compound ("ran and skipped and hopped"). The other options either have *more than one subject or more than one verb*.

14. B. Matthew was tall and shy, and Thomas was short and talkative.

A *simple sentence* is one which has *one subject and one verb*, though both the subject and verb can be compound. Linked by the conjunction "and", sentence B is the only compound sentence above because it links the first sentence "Matthew was tall and shy" with the second sentence "Thomas was short and talkative".

15. D. "There's a bus coming, so hurry up and cross the street!" yelled Bob to the old woman.

"There's" is the subject and verb of the sentence written as a contraction so the apostrophe is needed; a comma is needed before "so" because what follows it is a dependent clause which must be separated from the single sentence with a comma. When writing dialogue, the punctuation is included inside the quotation marks; in this case an exclamation is appropriate because Bob is warning the old woman to get out of the way of the oncoming bus; the use of the verb "yelled" is a clue that the statement by Bob is exclamatory.

16. C. It's a long to-do list she left for us today: make beds; wash breakfast dishes; go grocery shopping; do laundry; cook dinner; and read the twins a bedtime story.

"It's" is the subject and verb joined together in a contraction, so an apostrophe is needed. The sentence introduces a list, so it must be preceded by a colon; because the list is comprised of phrases instead of single words, a semicolon is needed to separate each item.

17. A. My room was a mess so my mom made me clean it before I was allowed to leave the house.

The use of the possessive pronoun "my" and the singular pronoun "I" indicates that the sentence is written from the first person perspective. "You" and "your" are second person; "her" or "him" are third person.

18. C. The president of France is meeting with President Obama later this week.

When referring to the "president of France", "president" is just a noun denoting his position, so it is not capitalized. In the case of "President Obama", "President" is the title by which he is addressed, so it is a proper noun and requires capitalization. The other options are incorrectly capitalized.

19. D. climb; creak

"Climb" is the proper spelling to denote ascending the stairs; "clime" refers to climate. "Creak" denotes a squeaky sound; "creek" denotes a stream or small moving waterway.

20. D. I will have completed

The FUTURE PERFECT TENSE indicates that an action will have been finished at some point in the future. This tense is formed with "will" plus "have" plus the past participle of the verb (which can be either regular or irregular in form). "By this time next summer" is the clue that lets you know the coursework will be done some time in the future.

21. A. assent; aide
The word "Assent" means approval, which is what the teacher wants to do to show encouragement to novice teacher who is currently her "aide" or assistance in the classroom. "Ascent" denotes a climb; "aid" is a verb denoting the action of helping.

22. D. No one has offered to let us use their home for the office's end-of-year picnic.
"No one", a singular pronoun, requires a singular verb, "has". "Us" is the objective case pronoun which is needed to follow the verb "to let"; "ourselves" is the reflexive case which is not needed in this sentence; "we" is subjective. "Their" shows possession of "home"; spelled "there", this word denotes location (e.g. here or there).

23. C. The tornado struck without warning and caused extensive damage.
Incorporating all of the information from the four sentences logically and concisely, option C is the best choice.

24. C. caused
"Caused" is the verb in this sentence; "Carrying" is the subject. Though it may look like a verb, it is actually a gerund (a verb acting as a noun) which is the subject. Deleting extraneous words will help see this, so let's rewrite the sentence in its most basic form: "Carrying caused her to throw out her back." This way it is clear to see that "carrying" is the subject, and is not a verb.

25. B. My eyelids drooping and my feet going numb, I thought his boring lecture would never end.
This sentence most clearly concisely conveys all of the information in the four above sentences; structure is parallel and no awkward or extraneous words are included.

26. D. Comets are balls of dust and ice, comprised of leftover materials that did not become planets during the formation of our solar system.
"Comets" (a plural subject requiring a plural verb) "are" "comprised of" (meaning: made up of) leftover materials that "did not" (in the past) become planets during the formation of "our" solar system.

27. B. Improvements in printing resulted in the production of newspapers, as well as England's more fully recognizing the singular concept of reading as a form of leisure; it was, of itself, a new industry.
The sentence is a compound sentence (two complete subject and verb phrases), so these should be separated by a comma after newspapers. The possession of recognition of the singular concept of reading by England needs to be shown with an apostrophe plus "s": "England's".

28. A. era
The Victorian Era is a two-word proper noun referring to a time period in history so "era" should be capitalized. The other words should not be capitalized.

29. C. coresponding
The correct spelling is *corresponding*.

30. D. market
"this demand" refers back to the "*market* (for cheaper literature)" in the last sentence of paragraph 2.

31. C. Working class boys who could not afford a penny a week often formed clubs that would share the cost, passing the flimsy booklets from reader to reader.
This sentence most clearly and concisely expresses the idea of book sharing amongst working boys who could not afford to spend a penny every week to buy the penny dreadfuls.

32. B. gothic

The word Gothic is a proper adjective referring to a specific genre of literature. None of the other words in this sentence should be capitalized.

33. D. The penny dreadfuls were influential since they were in the words of one commentator "the most alluring and low-priced form of escapist reading available to ordinary youth."

The independent clause "in the words of one commentator" needs to be set off by commas on either end; and since it is a direct quote, the last part of the sentence needs to be in quotation marks. The period at the end of the sentence needs to be inside the quotation marks.

34. B. novels

A noun is a person, place or thing. "Novels" is a plural noun which denotes a *thing* that can be read. "Serial" and "sensational" are adjectives; "generally" is an adverb.

35. D. greater

An adjective is a word which describes a noun. In this sentence, "greater" is an adjective describing *fear*. "Circulation" and "literature" are nouns; "however" is a pronoun.

36. C. Paragraph 3

Paragraph mentions that penny dreadfuls were often plagiarized versions of other popular literature at the time, so this would be the best place to add a sentence of supporting detail about this.

37. A. baptist

As the word identifies King's religion, "Baptist" should be capitalized.

38. A. His efforts to achieve racial equality in the United States, and his staunch public advocacy of civil rights are undoubtedly among the most important cultural contributions made to society in the last century.

Using parallel structure and no extraneous verbiage, option A is the most clear and concise of the versions.

39. D. I Have a Dream

"I Have a Dream" is the title of a speech and should therefore be put inside quotation marks.

40. B. Piece

In this sentence, "Piece" should be spelled *Peace*, as in harmony or an absence of fighting.

41. D. Metal

In this sentence, "Metal" should be spelled "Medal", as an award or honor, not "metal" as in a naturally occurring element or raw material.

42. C. This speech alienated many of his liberal allies in government who supported the war, but to his credit King never allowed politics to dictate the path of his noble works. (P. 3)

The phrase "to his credit" and the description of his works as "noble" provide clues that the author has a positive perspective about Martin Luther King and the role his activism played in American history.

43. C. No, because the passage is about King's public life and works, and information about his family would be irrelevant.

The focus of the passage is about King's work as a minister and activist, so details about his family are unrelated to this focus, and therefore should be left out.

44. C. "I am making pancakes for breakfast. Does anybody want some?" asked mom.

Only option C correctly includes sentence punctuation for quoted statements: punctuation for dialogue should be inside quotation marks, as is illustrated with mom asking if anyone wants pancakes; the question mark is within the quotation marks.

45. B. I woke up early that morning and began to do long-neglected household chores.

Option B contains two simple sentences, which when combined make a compound sentence:" I woke up early than morning" AND "I began to do long-neglected household chores."

46. D. A, C, E, D, B

The most logical progression of ideas is in option D. The topic of Disney's public persona is introduced, and is then contrasted with his treatment of people at work, and then the transformation of his persona from that of an American patriot to an imperialist. Finally, the paragraph is wrapped up with statements about the importance of his work and his current legacy in popular culture.

47. C. began to have

The sentence is discussing the contrast between Disney's private and public personas, stating that he *began to have* a public persona which was very different than the way he was in private.

48. A. You had better call and RSVP to the party right away before you forget.

Statements which show direct address, and use the pronoun "you" are referred to as the second person. Though the exclamation uses the pronoun you, it is a quoted statement, so it is really in the third person. Only choice A is an example of second person writing.

49. D. Parents are reminded to pick up their children from school promptly at 2:30.

Only D makes proper use of pronouns and their antecedents: in A, *novels* and *it* do not agree; in B, *everyone* is singular, so instead of *their*, the pronoun should be *him or her*; in C, *companies* and *it* do not agree.

50. C. Rice and beans, my favorite meal, reminds me of my native country Puerto Rico.

Choice C is the only sentence in which subject (*rice and beans/meal*) and verb (*reminds*) agree: in A, *one* and *have lived* do not agree; in B, *one* and *are going* do not agree; and in D, most (*of the milk* OR *it*) does not agree with *have gone*.

51. C. "You barely know him! How can she marry him?" was the worried mother's response at her teenager's announcement of marriage.

Sentence punctuation always is inside quotation marks; therefore, option C is punctuated correctly for dialogue.

52. A. "I have a dream", began Martin Luther King, Jr.

Second person uses the pronoun "you" or features direct address. Though punctuated incorrectly, it is clear that only the first sentence is not written in the second person; the use of "I" illustrates first person.

53. D. "Please remain seated while the seatbelt signs are illuminated." Came the announcement over the airplane's loud speaker system.

An Imperative statement is one which gives a command. Though punctuated incorrectly, it is clear that option D is imperative: the announcement is commanding the passengers to remain seated.

54. C. Excision

The prefix "ex" means out, so that is our clue here. "Excision" refers to a surgical procedure done to cut out something unwanted or unnecessary.

55. B. Colitis

The suffix "itis" is one which refers to inflammation, so "colitis" is an inflammation of the colon.

56. D. Melanoma

The suffix "oma" refers to a tumor or cancer, so "melanoma" refers to a cancer of the skin (coming from melanin, that which gives our skin its color). "Oncology" is the *study* of cancer, but it does not refer to cancer itself.

57. C. Rhinitis

The root "rhino" refers to the nose or nasal area, so "rhinitis" is an inflammation of the nasal passages.

58. A. Gastroenterology

The suffix "logy" refers to the study of some discipline or area, therefore gastroenterology is the study or examination of the gastrointestinal area of the body.

ADVANCED PRACTICE TEST: ENGLISH

1. C. Counterfeiting of American money is an enormous problem.

C is the best option as we are told that "The Treasury goes to extraordinary lengths to safeguard cash from counterfeiters."

2. B. Yet, despite all of these technological innovations, the race to stay ahead of savvy counterfeiters and their constantly changing counterfeiting techniques is a never-ending one.

B is the best as the main point of the passage is to emphasize the extent of counterfeiting and detail the technology used to counteract such constantly changing fraudulent activity.

3. C. Expository

An expository essay is one in which an idea is investigated and expounded upon, and an argument is set forth presenting evidence concerning that idea in a clear and concise manner. In this case the idea being investigated and expounded upon is anti-counterfeiting techniques.

4. A. A pamphlet for tourists visiting the United States Treasury

The style and specific subject matter all indicate that it is most likely from an informational pamphlet written for visitors to the Bureau of Engraving and Printing.

5. C. A letter from the US treasury Secretary to the President

A primary source document is one which was created and serves as a first-hand source of information or evidence about a particular time period. Only the personal letter would meet the criteria of a primary source.

6. D. Inherent

Technological sophistication is inherent, (or naturally found) in the making of American money, so much so that to call it "paper" does not fully reveal how complex a product it really is.

7. **A. In the Middle Ages, merchants an artisans formed groups called "guilds" to protect themselves and their trades.**

The first sentence is the topic sentence because it introduces the main idea of the paragraph.

8. **C. merchant guilds originated in the Middle Ages and became extremely popular, eventually leading to a sophisticated apprenticeship system.**

The guild system's origins and development is the main idea of the paragraph. The other options are too narrow to constitute a main idea.

9. **A. prior to the inception of guilds, merchants were susceptible to competition from lesser skilled craftsmen peddling inferior products or services.**

It can be inferred that if guilds were instituted, there must have been a need for merchants to safeguard themselves from threats to their livelihood.

10. **C. similar**

The sentence conveys to us that the spice, silk and wool dealers were similar tradesman to that of other merchants who had set up guilds.

11. **C. By that time,**

The passage introduces the inception of guilds and their development over time, chronologically. From the previous sentence, it is clear that guilds grew in popularity over the centuries, until towns like Florence had 50 guilds by the twelfth century. "By that time" most clearly states this increase and development over time.

12. **B. To criticize the American press for not taking responsibility for their actions**

Luce is clearly criticizing the press for not taking responsibility to disseminate enlightening information to the public, and instead are blaming the public for not asking for reading matter which is "tasteful and more illuminating".

13. **A. A newspaper editorial letter**

Given the paragraph's opinionated style and serious, critical tone, it most likely excerpted from a longer letter printed in the op/ed section of a newspaper.

14. **C. A diary entry**

The diary entry (which would likely provide firsthand thoughts, feelings and opinions about current life or world events as witnessed by the author) would qualify as a primary source document of evidence or information of a particular time period.

15. **D. enlightening**

Illuminating reading matter is that which would be enlightening and provide necessary information to the public.

16. **C. therefore**

Luce is using a cause and effect argument here, but she is questioning the excuse of the press to not do their job as a result of certain demands of the public, which would "therefore exonerate the American press for its failures to give the American people more tasteful and more illuminating reading matter".

17. **C. disapproval**

Luce clearly disapproves of the press and their practice of serving up a lack of news to the public, "on the grounds that, after all, "[they] have to give the people what they want or [they] will go out of business".

18. B. persuasive/argumentative

Luce utilizes several modes of writing here, but overall, she is critical of the American press, and is *arguing* that they are at fault for not giving the American public useful information or "illuminating reading matter".

19. B. The author has worked in the journalism industry

The author clearly has an understanding of the business of the media, as well as its public responsibility to inform citizens, so it can be concluded that she likely has worked in the journalism industry. None of the other statements can reasonably be concluded based on the content of the passage.

20. B. Football was played for decades on school campuses nationwide before the American Professional Football Association was formed in 1920, and then renamed the National Football League (or the NFL) two years later.

This statement adds additional information to the paragraph about the progression of the game of football in the US and therefore, appropriately concludes the paragraph. The other statements discuss topics not directly related to football, or add additional information that is slightly off topic.

21. A. however

The sentence is explaining that, despite the appearance of football as a sport on some college campuses, and annual scrimmages occurring at Yale, 25 years passed before it became a regular activity in college life. "However" shows this contrast best.

22. A. Rejection of the past and outmoded ideas

From the paragraph it is clear that modernism is mainly concerned with rejecting the ideas of the past -- like the science of the enlightenment, and old ideas about religion –and instead focusing on creating what was "New".

23. B. Basis

Pound's suggestion to "Make it new" was the basis, or *touchstone* of the Modernist movement's outlook and approach to interpreting the world and society.

24. D. Modernism had a profound impact on numerous aspects of life, and its values and perspectives still influence society in many positive ways today.

The author's description of Modernism's influence as being "positive" is clearly an opinion about the nature of the influence. The other statements are factually based, providing general information about the Modernist movement.

25. D. as well as

This sentence discusses all of the positive benefits that result from the continuation of the Olympic games in the present day, so "as well as" is the correct signal phrase to convey this idea, in a list form.

26. D. Detracted

The idea that allowing professional athletes to participate in the games would cause people to believe it "detracted" from the intentions of the original, is a negative notion, as it suggests that this would *take away from* the games, instead of adding something positive.

27. B. The Olympic games are the best example of humanity's physical prowess.

This statement is the opinion of the author, as there is no indication that this idea has been tested or proven in any way, but is simply what the author believes or feels.

28. C. Revulsion

The author uses words like "moldy smell" and "black hole" to describe his rented room in the inn, and "heartless" and "hideous" to describe the environment of London, adding that he "would rather even starve" than go out to find himself a meal in the "hellish town where a stranger might get trampled to death". These are very strong negative sentiments that clearly indicate his *revulsion* to the city.

29. B. A diary entry

The personal and frank tone that the author uses to describe his hotel room and his private fears about going out into the city of London for dinner suggest that this would have been written in a journal or diary.

30. D. An advertisement

A primary source document is one which was created from first-hand experience under a period of study of a particular event, moment in time, situation etc. A travel guide, diary entry and news editorial could all potentially be primary sources which chronicle one of the aforementioned. The only one that would likely NOT qualify as a primary source is the advertisement, as usually advertisements are meant to persuade one to engage in an experience, purchase a product or the like, and are often not completely based in personal experience and may not even be factual.

31. D. The author will not be traveling to London again.

It is clear that the author is unhappy with his lodging and finds London a generally disagreeable place, so it is likely that he would not travel to London again. The other statements are not reasonable conclusions which can be made from the content of the passage.

CPSIA information can be obtained
at www.ICGtesting.com
Printed in the USA
LVOW09s0920261117
557606LV00008BA/21/P

9 780996 870696